ADDRESSING THE SEXUAL RIGHTS OF OLDER PEOPLE

There is growing evidence that the sexual rights of older people are not being met. One reason, perhaps the main reason, relates to the way that old age is viewed. In many cultures, being old is associated with decline and disease, which positions older people as dependent and powerless. Furthermore, an absence of positive or celebratory discourses around older people's sexuality is particularly striking.

The book addresses a gap in research and policy. Using an adaptation of the Declaration of Sexual Rights from the World Association of Sexual Health, it provides readers with an innovative and evidence-based framework for achieving the sexual rights of older people. Drawing on interdisciplinary research, it explores the social locations of old age and its intersections with, for example, sexual orientation, gender identity, and intersex. Key themes include stigma, silencing, invisibility, prejudice, discrimination, and a lack of information, awareness, and understanding.

Addressing the Sexual Rights of Older People: Theory, Policy and Practice is a text for academics, health professionals, social professionals, service providers, and policymakers. It is a timely and insightful collection that suggests ways to apply the sexual rights framework, to raise awareness, and to engage communities in constructing strategies for reform.

Catherine Barrett is Director of Celebrate Ageing and The OPAL Institute, a national program promoting the sexual rights of older Australians.

Sharron Hinchliff is Senior Lecturer at the School of Nursing and Midwifery, University of Sheffield, where she leads the ageing, gender, and sexual health and well-being programme of research.

ADDRESSING THE SEXUAL RIGHTS OF OLDER PEOPLE

Theory, Policy and Practice

Edited by Catherine Barrett and Sharron Hinchliff

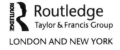

Routledge
Taylor & Francis Group

LONDON AND NEW YORK

First published 2018
by Routledge
2 Park Square, Milton Park, Abingdon, Oxon OX14 4RN

and by Routledge
711 Third Avenue, New York, NY 10017

Routledge is an imprint of the Taylor & Francis Group, an informa business

© 2018 Catherine Barrett and Sharron Hinchliff

British Library Cataloguing-in-Publication Data
A catalogue record for this book is available from the British Library

Library of Congress Cataloging-in-Publication Data
A catalog record for this book has been requested

ISBN: 978-1-138-18917-1 (hbk)
ISBN: 978-1-138-18918-8 (pbk)
ISBN: 978-1-315-64175-1 (ebk)

Typeset in Bembo
by Apex CoVantage, LLC

This book is dedicated to Delys Sargeant,
an early pioneer of sexual rights for older people.
And to Trevor Hinchliff and Carol Hinchliff,
with much love.

CONTENTS

EDITOR BIOGRAPHIES

Catherine Barrett has over 30 years' experience working with older people as a clinician, educator, researcher and capacity builder. Catherine established Australia's first Sexual Health and Ageing Program at La Trobe University, which included ground-breaking research on sexual narratives, sexual assault, sexually transmissible infections, and sexual and gender diversity. In 2016 Catherine established the OPAL Institute, a national program conducting research, developing policy and resourcing older people and service providers to address the sexual rights of older people. The OPAL Institute's first policies on *Sexuality in Residential Aged Care* and *Sexual Boundaries in Home Services* are being utilised by service providers to address sexual rights.

Sharron Hinchliff is a Senior Lecturer at the School of Nursing and Midwifery, University of Sheffield. She has been conducting research into gendered health for over 20 years. Sharron currently leads the ageing, gender, sexual health, and sexual well-being programme of research at the University, which examines the psychological, social, and cultural factors that influence health and healthcare. Her research is concerned with changing social attitudes towards older people, sex, and relationships, and it aims to improve professional healthcare practice in this area. She has published extensively for academic, clinical, and lay audiences. For further details, visit Sharron's website: www.sharronhinchliff.com

CONTRIBUTOR BIOGRAPHIES

Graham Brown is a Senior Research Fellow at the Australian Research Centre in Sex, Health and Society at La Trobe University. Graham has worked in STI and HIV community-based health promotion and research for 20 years. He has a particular interest in the partnership of health services, community-based organisations, research and policy in enhancing the sexual health and rights of communities. Graham is a past President of the Australian Federation of AIDS Organisations and continues to serve on a number of State and National BBV and STI-related health promotion and policy committees.

Raffaella Ferrero Camoletto is Associate Professor in Sociology of Culture at the Department of Cultures, Politics and Society of the University of Turin, Italy. She has been extensively working on gender and (hetero)sexualities, with a focus on the medicalization of male sexuality. Among her recent research projects are "Beyond a naturalised masculinity? Making sense of the medicalisation of male sexuality" (2010–2016) and "Ageless sex? Questioning active ageing in the Viagra era" (2016-ongoing). Among her recent publications are *Le fragilità del sesso forte. Medicalizzare la sessualità*, Mimesis, Roma (2016, with C. Bertone); *Medicalizing male underperformance: expert discourses on male sexual health in Italy*, Salute e Società, XIV, n.1, 183–205 (2015, with C.Bertone, F.Salis); and *Italians (should) do it better? Medicalization and the disempowering of intimacy*, in *Modern Italy*, Vol. 17, No. 4, 433–448 (2012, with Bertone C.).

Laura Hurd Clarke is a Professor in the School of Kinesiology at the University of British Columbia in Vancouver, Canada. Her research interests lie in the areas of ageing, ageism, gender, and the body. To date, her work has explored older men's and women's body image, experiences of chronic conditions and disability, use of anti-ageing practices and products, perceptions of assistive technologies, and engagement in self-care and physical activity.

Loree Cook-Daniels has been working on both LGBT and ageing issues since 1974. In the 1990s she was a primary staff person for the National Center on Elder Abuse. She founded the Transgender Aging Network in 1998, and in 2000 became the Policy and Program Director for FORGE, a 23-year-old national transgender and SOFFA (Significant Others, Friends, Family, and Allies) organization that specializes in transgender ageing and victims of violence. Formerly a contributing editor for the *Victimization of the Elderly and Disabled*, she has also authored numerous book chapters, articles and tip sheets on LGBT and trans ageing issues. FORGE's Transgender Aging Network was a founding partner in the National Resource Center on LGBT Aging and remains its primary transgender expert. She holds a B.A. in Women's Studies and History, an M.S. in Conflict Management, and a Graduate Certificate in Trauma Counseling.

Pauline Crameri is the co-ordinator of Val's LGBTI Ageing and Aged Care – a program that seeks to improve the health, well-being and visibility of older LGBTI Australians through research, resource development and building the capacity of services to become LGBTI aware and inclusive. Val's is part of Gay and Lesbian Health Victoria at the Australian Centre in Sex, Health and Society, La Trobe University, Melbourne, Australia. Pauline has more than 20 years' experience in aged care including research, community aged care assessment, care planning and project management, and aged care planning. Pauline has practical experience in LGBTI inclusive service development and delivery and lead a service to achieve the first Rainbow Tick accreditation.

Dr Bianca Fileborn is a Lecturer in Criminology in the School of Social Sciences, at the University of New South Wales. Her work is broadly concerned with interrogating the intersections of identity, space, place, culture and experiences of violence. In particular, her current work focuses on sexual violence and harassment. She is also interested in concepts of justice, and particularly informal, innovative, and transformative justice. Bianca's recent work includes an examination of unwanted sexual attention and sexual violence in licensed venues; experiences, impacts and justice responses to street harassment; sexuality and ageing; policing and LGBTIQ+ young people; and the sexual assault of older women. Her sole-authored monograph, 'Reclaiming the Night-Time Economy: Unwanted Sexual Attention in Pubs and Clubs', was published by Palgrave in 2016.

M. Morgan Holmes is Full Professor and Graduate Programme Director in Sociology at Wilfrid Laurier University in Waterloo, Canada, where she teaches courses in critical disability studies and the social science of medicine. Currently editing a special collection for the *Canadian Journal of Disability Studies* on disability and sexuality, Morgan is also the editor of the only collection of international scholarship on Intersex (*Critical Intersex*, Ashgate Press, 2011) and is the author of *Intersex: A Perilous Difference* (Susquehanna, 2008). Morgan is currently working on a monograph on cancer screening and the production of cancer as an industry. Morgan recently co-authored, with Eddie Ing, a major human rights report on the needs for intersex children and adults to be included in gender-based protection laws in Canada; the report has been submitted to the office of the Prime Minister through the Just Society Committee at EGALE.

Dr Hans Wiggo Kristiansen is a social anthropologist currently working as senior advisor at Oslo Church City Mission. He has worked as a researcher at Norwegian Social Research (NOVA) and the University of Oslo and has published and coedited several books, research reports, chapters and journal articles on living conditions, life narratives and ageing among LGBT people in Norway. His research has been funded by the Research Council of Norway.

J.R. Latham is an Honorary Fellow in Screen and Cultural Studies at The University of Melbourne, Australia. His research explores how trans and intersex people experience sex, gender, embodiment and sexuality on their own terms, and the manifest tensions between self-determination and clinical practices of medicine. His work has been published in *Aesthetic Plastic Surgery,* the *Australasian Journal on Ageing, Feminist Theory, Sexualities* and *Studies in Gender and Sexuality.* In 2016, Latham was co-winner of the Symonds Prize for the essay "Making and Treating Trans Problems: The Ontological Politics of Clinical Practices" and his doctoral research received the Nancy Millis University Medal from La Trobe University. Visit www.jrlatham.com

June Lowe is Chair of GRAI (GLBTI Rights in Ageing Inc.), a community-based nongovernmental organisation supporting the rights and well-being of LGBTI elders in Western Australia (WA). June has been a social activist since the 1980s, working on environmental and social justice issues, including gay rights law reform in WA in 2001. She is intrigued by social change and the role we all play in shaping it, and takes heart at the remarkable progress that has been achieved, locally and globally, in healing the social stigma around LGBTI identity.

Through her work with GRAI, June has taken a multi-level approach to create safe ageing environments for LGBTI elders, including law reform advocacy, research on LGBTI ageing, aged sector education, and community building. She contributes to government enquiries regarding LGBTI elders' needs and is a member of National LGBTI Ageing and Aged Care Strategy Working Group. She also coordinates and delivers LGBTI inclusivity training for aged care providers and is a frequent speaker at conferences and workshops. This work is informed and enriched by her direct engagement with LGBTI elders: organising numerous initiatives to strengthen social cohesion within the community, including individual support, group workshops, social activities and forays into LGBTI intergenerational projects.

Anthony Lyons is Associate Professor in the Australian Research Centre in Sex, Health and Society (ARCSHS) at La Trobe University. Anthony specialises in the areas of sexual health and mental health. He works with a range of populations, including older people, individuals living with HIV, and people who identify as lesbian, gay, bisexual, or transgender. His research has attracted funding from a wide variety of sources, including research councils, governments, foundations, and non-profit organisations. His work is also regularly used to inform evidence-based policy and practice. Anthony has published 81 scholarly works, including journal articles, books, and book chapters. His work has also attracted media attention around the world, such as in the *New York Times*, *The Huffington Post*, *New Zealand Herald*, ABC radio, *The Age*, and the *Sydney Morning Herald*.

Sue Malta is a Research Fellow at the National Ageing Research Institute, where she works on projects involving the care and well-being of older adults. She is a sociologist with research interests in ageing, love and sexuality in heterosexual and diverse populations, social connection/isolation and carers, amongst others. Her PhD investigated love, sex and intimacy in new late-life romantic relationships, online and offline. Sue also works at the School of Population and Global Health, University of Melbourne, on a project involving sexual health and ageing; and is an Adjunct Research Fellow at Swinburne University, where she collaborates on projects addressing sexual health promotion and ageing. She is a collaborator on the La Trobe University project *Sex, Age & Me* and is on the Steering Committee for the COTA Vic/Transgender Vic project *Supporting Older Trans and Gender Diverse Victorians to Plan for End of Life*. As an early career researcher she has published widely and in 2012 contributed a chapter entitled "Using online methods to interview older adults about their romantic and sexual relationships" in *Researching Later Life and Ageing – Expanding Qualitative Research Horizons* published by Palgrave. She is a member of AAG, TASA and the Sexual Health Society of Victoria.

Michael Munson is the co-founder and Executive Director of FORGE, an organization focused on improving the lives of transgender individuals by building stronger connections, providing resources, and empowering growth through knowledge. FORGE is a national training and technical assistance provider funded through the Department of Justice, Office on Violence Against Women and the Office for Victims of Crime. Michael's educational background is in psychology, with an emphasis on trauma-informed care and non-traditional healing modalities. His work on violence against transgender and non-binary individuals stresses the intersectionality between complex components of identity, experience, and societal constructs that can both spur violence as well as catalyze healing for individuals and communities. He is passionate about engaging professionals to embrace these complexities and learn key skills to better serve their clients/constituents.

Karen A. Roberto is a University Distinguished Professor, Director of the Institute for Society, Culture and Environment Center and Senior Fellow at the Center for Gerontology at Virginia Polytechnic Institute and State University. She holds secondary appointments in the Department of Internal Medicine and the Department of Psychiatry and Behavioral Medicine at the Virginia Tech Carilion School of Medicine. Her research focuses on health and social support in late life and includes studies of the health of rural older women, family relationships and caregiving, and elder abuse. Much of Karen's research relies on the construction of surveys for use with community-based samples, combines quantitative and qualitative methodologies, and often includes interviews with older adults, family members, and formal service providers. She has published over 175 scholarly articles and book chapters and is editor/author of 11 books. Karen is a fellow of the American Psychological Association, the Gerontological Society of America, the Association for Gerontology in Higher Education, and the National Council on Family Relations. She is the recipient of the Gerontological Society of America Behavioral and Social Sciences Distinguished Mentorship Award and the Virginia Tech Alumni Award for Excellence in Research.

Summer Roberts is an Assistant Professor of Sociology at the University of South Carolina, Beaufort. Her research and teaching focus on intersections of ageing and gender from a social psychological perspective. Summer's recent publications include an article examining gender differences in online dating for middle-aged and older adults in the *Journal of Family Issues* and another on the use of identity work by members of a lifelong learning institute in the *Journal of Gerontology: Social Sciences*. Her ongoing in-depth interview research examines how social location, residential history, and planning for the future relate to older adults' perspectives on the self as ageing successfully. Over the past year, Summer has worked with faculty in sociology, psychology, human services, and nursing to develop a Gerontology Certificate program at USCB in order to prepare students for better serving the region, one-quarter of which consists of adults aged 65 and older.

Linn J. Sandberg is Assistant Professor and Lecturer in Gender Studies at Stockholm University and Södertörn University College, Sweden. Her work focuses on the intersections of gender, sexuality and ageing and makes dialogues between gender and sexualities studies and critical cultural gerontology. Linn's previous research on masculinity, sexuality and ageing, emerging from her doctoral dissertation, has been published in international peer-reviewed journals such as *Men and Masculinities*, *Sexualities*, and *International Journal of Aging and Later Life*. She is the author of chapters on sex and sexuality in later life in the volumes *The Routledge Handbook of Cultural Gerontology* (eds. Twigg & Martin, 2015), *Introducing the New Sexualities Studies* (eds. Fischer & Seidman, 2016) and *Ageing and Everyday Life: Materialities and Embodiments* (ed. Katz, forthcoming). Currently she is the principal investigator of a research project on Alzheimer's disease, sexuality, intimacy and coupledom.

Rachel Thorpe is a Research Fellow at the Australian Research Centre in Sex, Health and Society at La Trobe University, Australia. Her doctoral work focused upon women's experiences of sexuality, relationships and appearance in later life. Her research interests include: how people make sense of and negotiate bodily ageing, ageing and generational change, and living with chronic illness. She has previously undertaken research in the areas of living with HIV, use of complementary medicines and the regulation of assisted reproductive technologies.

Emily Wentzell is an Associate Professor in the University of Iowa Department of Anthropology and director of the University of Iowa International Studies Program. Her research combines approaches from medical anthropology, gender studies, and science and technology studies to examine sexual health interventions' gendered social consequences across the life course, focusing on Mexico and the U.S.

Sue Westwood is a feminist socio-legal and social gerontology scholar. She is a Lecturer in Law at Keele University, UK, where she has designed a new course entitled 'Law and the Older Person', and is the Law School Lead for Technology Enhanced Learning. Sue's research focuses on (a) ageing, gender and sexuality in regulatory contexts; (b) law's operation in closed care spaces; and (c) the regulation of death and dying, particularly in older age. She is a member of the following research clusters at Keele: Healthcare Law and Bioethics (HLB); Private Law: Theory and Practice (PLTP); Social Justice and Human Rights (SJHR); Keele Centre for Ageing Research (KCAR). Sue's book, *Ageing, Gender and Sexuality: Equality in later life*, won the Socio-Legal Studies Association's Early Career Prize for 2017. In collaboration with Elizabeth Price (University of Hull), Sue has also co-edited a collection published by Routledge: *Lesbian, Gay, Bisexual and Trans* Individuals Living with Dementia: Concepts, practice and rights*. She is a member of the Socio-Legal Studies Association, the Law and Society Association, and the British Society of Gerontology.

FOREWORD

The population of our world continues to increase and over the forthcoming decades there will be significant changes to the age distribution within the population. In 2015, the United Nations predicted that the world population of 7.3 billion will rise to 9.7 billion by 2050 and to 11.2 billion by 2100. The number of persons aged 60 or above is expected to more than double by 2050 and more than triple by 2100. Research into the sexual health and the overall well-being of older people (however this is defined) has unfortunately been neglected until relatively recently.

Sharron Hinchliff, a social and health psychologist has established a portfolio of research in the fields of sexual and reproductive health, ageing and gender and her work features in many of the lectures that I have delivered over many years. Since working at the Sheffield Institute for Studies on Ageing, and then at the School of Nursing and Midwifery (both at the University of Sheffield) Sharron has developed her expertise in these diverse and important subject areas and it has been a privilege to be able to collaborate with Sharron on several projects during my time working in Sheffield. Catherine Barrett began addressing the sexual rights of older people over 20 years ago as a nurse working in aged care. Catherine went on to establish a Sexual Health and Ageing research program at La Trobe University and most recently launched the OPAL Institute – an Australian based program addressing the sexual rights of older people.

The sexual health needs of older people have also featured in a number of projects led by Gunta Lazdane, Regional Advisor on Sexual Reproductive Health Rights at the WHO Europe office in Copenhagen. The invitation and encouragement to participate in a number of these events have also been instrumental to me, and other professionals, in highlighting the vast importance of this previously neglected field within medicine and health care generally. The impact has been substantial and led me to speak about Relationships, Ageing and Equality as the topic of my final

Presidential lecture for the World Association for Sexual Health (WAS) congress in Prague, 2017.

In recent decades there has been a culture of facilitating movement away from discrimination of minority populations often as a consequence of sustained and strong advocacy by professionals and other interested individuals and groups. This has gone some way towards reducing the discrimination of many recognised – and in some countries protected – minority groups within society. These include, but are not exclusively with regard to, sexual orientation, gender identity, ethnicity, religion, race, wealth, health and younger age. The protection and promotion of rights of all persons belonging to any of these minority groups has substantially reduced the overall number of violations of the many rights that most of us take for granted. However, each of these minority groups may also co-exist within people of older age and if discrimination is not identified within this group of people generally, there remains the risk of multiple discrimination occurring in this often hidden group of people within society.

Within contemporary societies and cultures, people of older age may remain silent and forgotten about in many social environments. The opportunities to express and share their experiences with regard to how they experience discrimination especially of a sexual nature are often limited or non-existent. This discrimination may reflect neglect rather than deliberate attempts to inflict harm or embarrassment to individuals but is albeit still a source of stigma to individuals, couples and carers. Regardless of any intent, the impact and effects of any type or variation of discrimination is often unpredictable for an individual but will usually be experienced as harmful and with significant impact on the emotional, mental and physical well-being for the individual.

It is reassuring that there is an increasing number of researchers and advocates who give strong priority to understanding the experiences and concerns for older people. Sadly, this may be too late to offer advantage for some of the people facing significant challenges from health and social care systems and from society in general. All of us can start to make change by making this a topic that is thought about and talked about in all parts of our life and certainly well beyond the workplace.

So, it was with great pleasure to receive the invitation to write the foreword to this innovative and creative book by two distinguished authors in the field. Catherine and Sharron have brought together a number of colleagues with vast expertise on this topic and who collectively deliver authoritative information and signposting in this developing field of academic, clinical and educational importance. The authors deliver a multitude of resources from their diverse breadth of experience of people from minority groups within society and I commend this credible book to the readership.

From a practical perspective, how can we deal effectively with ensuring that the issue of sexual rights of older people is addressed adequately as this group become an increasing proportion of the overall population and are no longer a minority group? Society can ill afford to or be allowed to neglect and ignore the basic human rights of older people. It could be argued that collectively they will be in a position of greater strength with a stronger voice through democratic election and other means to ensure that there can be demands for changes in provision of social and health care. My sense is that it could be some time before this will become well-established even in the most contemporary of Western societies. It is likely that it will remain some time yet before older persons will command the same respect expected by the younger members of society who maintain a much stronger representation and awareness. How can we enable authority for this heterogeneous group of individuals within our communities to ensure that the intimate and sexual needs of every single person is respected, enabled and preserved? I would like to suggest that there are at least three important contributors to ensuring that this can happen.

First is the publication of this book that provides an ideal starting point by opening up opportunities for clinicians and educators to consider many of the important issues that may be experienced by the increasing number of older people within the population. As a consequence, we can try to ensure that society is educated, informed and enabled to reach a more informed position that asks about, listens to and as a consequence appreciates the sexual aspirations and needs of people of older age. I suggest that we allow free expression of diversity inherent within older people, recognising that much of this diversity is the same as within society as a whole. As such it is not exclusively related to the ageing process itself however much this may be conveniently attributed by some who remain content to ignore their own prejudices and discrimination.

Second is an appreciation of the impact of ensuring the respect, protection and fulfilment of all human rights. The adverse impact of any violation of human rights means that human rights are now considered essential for maintaining optimum public health and social justice. Within the World Association for Sexual Health (WAS), it is our statement that despite the absence of the use of the term sexual rights in the new 2030 Agenda for Sustainable Development adopted by the United Nations in 2015, the clear commitment to ensuring universal access to sexual and reproductive health care services and the universal respect for human rights and human dignity and the rule of law, justice, equality and non-discrimination means that sexual rights should now be well protected within society (Kismodi et al. 2017).

Third could be an open acknowledgement that sexual rights are an essential component of human rights. With the adoption of the revised WAS Declaration of Sexual Rights in 2015 it is crucial to appreciate that no new human rights standards were created and that existing rights were strengthened by reference to official texts, decisions and interpretations of legally codified human rights that related to sexuality and sexual health. This was achieved by a thorough review of the work of national, regional and international human rights and legislative bodies.

This book emphasises the general and the specific needs and rights of the ageing population and refers to these within the context of the revised WAS Declaration of Sexual Rights. The interpretation of the Declaration of Sexual Rights by the authors as it can be best applied to ageing persons as well as to other specific minority groups of people is to be welcomed and I offer my strong endorsement of such. Our statement within WAS is clear and that is the reaffirmation of sexual health and rights must extend to all stages of the life cycle for human beings. Each stage of life may have specific needs that must be addressed and accommodated. No person who has sexual needs should be denied the opportunity to experience those needs and that includes exclusion of those needs on the grounds of older age. These needs can be multiple and complex with an example being a recently widowed seventy-eight-year young black bisexual man living in Senegal with diabetes mellitus. He develops a prolonged grief response and depression to the death of his wife and also suffers with the complications of his diabetes with sensory loss neuropathy, problems of mobility and is unable to continue to live independently. When he meets a man in the care home with whom he wishes to establish intimate relationships, he may consider seeking help for long-standing erectile dysfunction (another complication of the diabetes and a normal consequence of ageing) from his medical practitioner. He is uncertain about the response he will receive from his physician. Further, he has yet to learn that some oral tablet treatments to improve erectile function – if prescribed and affordable – may interact and exacerbate normal side effects of these agents as the consequence of him being prescribed pharmacological treatments for his long standing HIV positive status.

The WAS states categorically that sexual autonomy and bodily integrity of older people should be respected and protected, and this is especially important for those who live in elderly care homes and institutions. In these circumstances, we advocate that special and specific measures should be taken to ensure the protection of older people from all forms of neglect, trauma, violence and coercion.

I anticipate that this book will inspire readers to reflect and advocate successfully for the recognition of the often multiple minority stressors experienced by those living into their older years of life. We must ensure that any discrimination that becomes recognised as such shall lead to immediate action to ensure the discrimination will cease. The sexual health and well-being, the sexual rights and the human rights for this group of people within our society should be unequivocally championed by all of us whilst we are able to take such action.

Professor Kevan Wylie MD FRCP FRSPH
Sexual Medicine, Neurosciences, University of Sheffield;
President, World Association for Sexual Health (2012-2017)

Reference

Kismodi E, Corona E, Maticka-Tindall E, Rubio-Aurioles E, Coleman E. (2017) 'Sexual Rights as Human Rights: A Guide for the WAS Declaration of Sexual Rights', *International Journal of Sexual Health,* Volume 29 (in press).

ACKNOWLEDGEMENTS

We would like to acknowledge the growing number of researchers, academics, clinicians, and advocates who are fighting for recognition of the sexual rights of older people. In particular, the contributors to the chapters of this book from whom we have learned so much about the rich diversity of older people, as each author has addressed central questions about ageing, sexuality, and rights. We would like to thank Professor Kevan Wylie, President of the World Association for Sexual Health (WAS), for writing the Foreword, and the WAS team for ensuring that their Declaration of Sexual Rights is inclusive of all people. Thanks also to the team at Routledge, in particular Grace McInnes, Carolina Antunes, and Louisa Vahtrick, and Autumn Spalding at Apex CoVantage for encouragement, guidance, and overall support.

1

INTRODUCTION TO THE SEXUAL RIGHTS OF OLDER PEOPLE

Sharron Hinchliff and Catherine Barrett

Introduction

Sexual rights are simply human rights as applied to sexuality (Lenoir & Dortch 2011) and, as Shirin Heidari notes, they are subject to 'power relations in both the private and public domains' and always politically motivated (Heidari 2015). Sexual rights are culturally, socially, and historically situated yet globally they have been applied predominantly in relation to young people. There are many reasons for this, including young people being most at risk of sexual violations and disease, but also the assumption that sexuality does not apply to older people: as though, based on old age, issues related to sexual health, sexual well-being, sexual orientation, and gender identity simply do not matter. Viewing sexual rights within the framework of young people reflects the neglect of older people from the area of sexual and reproductive health overall. This collection of original essays takes sexual rights in a different direction by exploring the sexual rights of people aged 65 and older. Using an adaptation of the working definition from the World Health Organization (WHO) of sexuality as a 'central aspect of being human' that encompasses sex, sexual orientation, gender identities and roles, intimacy, pleasure, and eroticism (World Health Organization 2006), the book calls for a shift in how the sexuality of older people is viewed and approached. It not only addresses a gap in the literature – to the best of our knowledge this academic text is the first to examine older people's sexual rights – but it also moves beyond the heterosexual, lesbian, gay, and bisexual divide to incorporate transgender and intersex issues. We seek to provide readers with an innovative framework for addressing the sexual rights of older people: one which is both evidence-based and applicable to professional practice.

In this chapter we outline our rationale for why a sexual rights framework for older people is needed now. We then discuss the concepts and arguments that are pivotal to providing context to sexuality and ageing. We end by presenting an overview of the chapters that form this collection, each written by leading authors in their field, based in various geographical locations, and which present a range of theoretical perspectives. Individually, the chapters provide insight into specific sexually-related topics to deepen our understanding of them. Collectively, the chapters form a rights-based approach that will be useful to academics, health and social professionals, service providers, and policy-makers who work in the ageing and sexuality fields.

Why a sexual rights framework is needed now

Older people in contemporary Western societies have grown up during periods of significant social change. They have lived through, and participated in, grassroots movements (e.g. feminism and gay rights) that have altered social attitudes and transformed government policies. They have observed advances in medicine, science, and technology that have improved many people's quality of life and increased their life expectancy. But they have also experienced a time when sexuality was not openly discussed, when the menopause was taboo, and sexual activity outside of a marital relationship was frowned upon, particularly for women. Furthermore, those who did not conform to heterosexual and gender binary norms could risk being subjected to 'cure' therapies or imprisonment.

The way that sexuality, in its broadest sense, is understood and experienced is influenced by our social and cultural location. Life expectancy differs markedly from country to country (as an example, life expectancy at birth ranges from 50 years in Sierra Leone to 55 years in Somalia to 68 years in India and 83 years in Switzerland: World Health Organization 2016), influenced predominantly by war, disease, and accessible health care, so disparities between what we understand 'old' to mean exist globally. Attitudes toward lesbian, gay, bisexual, transgender, and intersex (LGBTI) people vary widely. In Iran, for example, it is against the law to be a gay man but not to be male-to-female transgender; the former is punished by death or imprisonment. These factors are important to consider in any sexual rights framework aimed at older people. As 'contexts of sexuality', they have an impact on the policies for, and resources available to, people in older age, which in turn can have a powerful influence on an individual's knowledge, beliefs, and behaviours, and capacity to assert their sexual rights. For example, a study carried out by Kaighobadi et al. (2014) of black South African men who had sex with men found that the older participants (the highest age was 40) did not perceive themselves to be at risk of sexually contracted HIV because HIV health promotion was aimed solely at their younger counterparts (Kaighobadi et al. 2014).[1]

A lot has changed over the past 50 years, ensuring that an individual's experience of being old today is very different from that of their parents. Global human rights have been established to help protect people from inequalities based on age, sexuality, gender, race, and socio-economic status (see Chapter 2). And shifts in social attitudes have been observed particularly around 'who can have sex with whom'.

Indeed, surveys such as the *British Social Attitudes* (Park et al. 2008) demonstrate that people are more tolerant of sexual activity outside of a married relationship: a shift that older people themselves are embracing as many choose to 'live apart together' rather than relinquish their own homes and independence during a newly formed intimate relationship (Karlsson & Borrell 2005).

Progressions in science have also influenced the change in what it means to be an older person today (e.g. through improving health in later life), and the inter-relationship between science and culture is very clear to see in the area of sexuality. Looking at history always provides an interesting insight. For example, from the 1960s onwards women were informed by medical experts that hormone therapy would 'restore' the femininity, sexual desire, and sexual attractiveness they had 'lost' as a result of the menopause and their declining levels of oestrogen (see Reuben 1970). This position reflected the dominant socio-cultural view of women at the time, and it is apt at this point to remember the words of Joy Webster Barbre that "Science does not stand outside of culture; it is part of the culture within which it exists" (Barbre 1998, p. 250). It also served the interest of pharmaceutical companies, and thus can be considered to constitute the beginning of the medicalisation of sex as we currently know it. The implications of a 'hormone-ized body' (Marshall & Katz 2006) continue to be seen today as the focus on retaining sexual desire and desirability at *all* stages of the life-course turns sexual agency into an expectation which, in itself, may become a pressure to conform. More recently, the development of 'sexuopharmaceuticals' (Potts & Tiefer 2006) ensures that (some) people can continue to be sexually active even though they experience sexual difficulties associated with advancing age. Shifts such as these share an intimate relationship with the view that sexual activity is something we all are interested in, a natural act (Tiefer 1995), and one that has benefits for health and well-being. Indeed, the latter perspective gained traction over the 20th century as (heterosexual) sex was slowly uncoupled from reproduction (Hawkes 1996). And, in the contemporary world, is increasingly applied to older people. We return to the biomedicalisation of ageing sexuality in the following sections.

Evidence of change can also be seen in the large number of surveys that now collect data on the extent and range of sexual activities older people engage in. They also have also begun to acknowledge that older people may be in same-sex relation-ships. Two striking examples from the UK include the *English Longitudinal Study of Ageing*, which included questions about sexual activities and intimate relation-ships for the first time in Wave 6 (2012–2013) -10 years after Wave 1 (2002) – and the *National Survey of Sexual Attitudes and Lifestyle*, which recruited participants up to age 74 in their third survey (2010–2012) - 20 years after the survey began in 1990. That these well-established major surveys altered their recruitment to include older people, or amended their focus to explore sex and intimacy, demonstrates a shift in social attitudes towards older people's relationships and sexual activity. Until recently, the assumption that older people were not sexually active, or if they were it was a private topic and they would not take part in research, was widespread and prevented progression in this area of research (Gott & Hinchliff 2003). As the evidence base has grown, so has the recognition of the sexual health needs of older adults. The WHO has made it clear that it views sexual health as a life-long concern, and we are now seeing the mention of older adults in national sexual health policy and guidelines for clinical practice and service provision (e.g. *A Framework for Sexual Health Improvement in England*: Department of Health 2013). This is a recent shift, occurring since the turn of the millennium and mainly in Western countries: it is a much-needed change. Consider the following example:

> Around diabetes and blood pressure say a man in his 40s, I might warn him and say 'this can have an effect on your sex drive'. . . . I might not mention it to a man in his 70s.
>
> *(Gott, Hinchliff & Galena 2004, p. 2097)*

The above scenario was described by a general practitioner[2] who took part in a research project that explored the management of sexual health within primary care. It is thus an instance of actual professional practice, and it is one of many. There is growing evidence that the sexual rights of older people are not being met on many levels. One reason, perhaps the *main* reason, connects with the way that older people are viewed. In Western societies, older age tends to be associated with decline, frailty, and disease – characteristics that are rarely associated with young people – and this construction of the older person positions them as dependent (e.g. on others for care), powerless, and highly vulnerable. Negative stereotypes of ageing such as these can be damaging, not only influencing the way that older people are viewed but also the resources that are made available to, and for, them.

Supporting older people's sexuality

There is evidence that age-related stereotypes can impact an older person's own behaviours as well as the way older people are responded to by others. Researchers have identified that older people who experience sexual difficulties do not always seek professional help, and one reason is the fear of being judged negatively for expressing an interest in sex 'at their age'. Another involves assuming that the sexual difficulty is age-related and therefore nothing can be done to help (see Hinchliff & Gott 2011 for a review of the literature). Research has also highlighted that older lesbians and gay men who require general health care tend not to disclose their sexual orientation to health and social professionals, arguing that a lifetime of prejudice and discrimination have affected their willingness to be open when accessing mainstream health and social services (see Chapter 5). Similarly, the third *National Survey of Sexual Attitudes and Lifestyles* (NATSAL 3) – the largest and most comprehensive survey of its kind in Britain – found that older women were less likely to report sexual assault (self-defined by the participants when asked about 'sex against their will') than younger women. The survey did not collect data on why this was the case, but the authors concluded that there was a need to 'de-stigmatise' the reporting of sexual assault for all women (Macdowall et al. 2013). We need to bear in mind that the survey asked about sex against their will since the age of 13 years, and for women the last occurrence ranged from 5–40 years ago. Older women may therefore have reported sex against their will that occurred during their younger years. Furthermore, it is possible that a cohort effect exists, and young women were more likely to report a sexual assault because they have had more opportunities to do so, as sexual assault has become more recognised over time. These are important points to consider, and the nuances around the sexual assault of older women are interrogated in Chapter 8.

The reasons why older people may be reluctant to seek help for sexually-related issues, to report a sexual crime, or to disclose their sexual orientation or gender identity to health and social professionals again should be understood in a socio-cultural context. Calasanti and Slevin (2006) have argued that older people often experience a loss of power, in terms of authority and autonomy, which is related to the structuring of age relations in the society where they live. Minichiello, Browne and Kendig (2000, p. 272), from their qualitative study of the meaning and experience of ageism for older Australians, made a similar point and introduced the concept of 'accommodated ageing' where "Older people may live their lives according to a philosophy of not making waves", which influences how they deal with ageism and their feelings of 'powerlessness' to challenge what happens to them.

The absence of positive or celebratory discourses around older people's sexuality can present a particular challenge for those who lose autonomy from disease or disability and find themselves dependent on others, who may be unsupportive of older people's sexuality. Clearly, older people are not always viewed as sexual beings; their sexual and intimacy needs often go unrecognised as assumptions are made about the nature of their interpersonal relationships. This is complicated by the actuality that as we get older our physical health can worsen, and our cognitive capacity may reduce. The argument may follow that an older person has health concerns to prioritise and so sexual health and well-being are not important to them. Although this might be applicable to some (e.g. those who experience disability and illness that interfere with sex and intimacy by imposing physical limitations that affect the sexual positions they can hold), it is not applicable to all.

As touched upon already, a lack of awareness and an absence of resources due to restrictive social attitudes can mean that health and social professionals do not always provide appropriate support for older people's sexuality issues. The WHO (2015) report *Sexual Health, Human Rights and the Law* asserts that the denial of access to education and services, a lack of protection from discrimination, and the non-protection of privacy and confidentiality within health and social care settings can negatively impact health and well-being. When older people are positioned outside of a sexual rights framework, they do not receive the care and support required for their sexually-related needs. We return to this issue in Chapter 12, where we describe strategies for change in the area of older people and sexual rights.

A sexual rights framework for older people is needed now, not only for the reasons discussed here but also for the reasons outlined in the chapters that make up this collection. As imperatives to 'age well' through remaining in good health and thus to be a 'virtuous' citizen are increasingly imposed, it is likely that future cohorts of older people will have different expectations of health and social care. Indeed, significant changes in the ways that being 'old', alongside being an older person with an interest in sex and intimacy, or being old and gay, have been observed over the past 50 years. We therefore need to be mindful that certain perspectives may gain prominence, become mainstream, and continue to shape what it means to be 'old'. One such issue is the current focus on the benefits of sexual activity for ageing health and well-being, which we now turn our attention to.

The medicalisation of sex and the 'sexy oldie'

The shift to recognising the sexual agency of older people has taken place over a short period of time. No doubt influenced, in part, by the sexualisation of culture – where increasing attention is focused on sexual activity and sexual appearance by the media, the fashion and music industries, and manufacturers that operate within this framework to sell their products – the sexual subjectivities of older people are increasingly visible and acknowledged. Indeed, it is only since the end of the 20th century that changes in the way that the sexual and intimate relationships of older people were observed in Western popular media. Previously, older people were denied any romantic attachments, but television advertisements began to create narratives that broke away from the predominant (and stereotypical) ways that they were previously portrayed (e.g. as the grey-haired, passive grandparent) (Williams et al. 2007; Vares 2009). There was also a disconnection from the type of sexually-related content presented in television dramas and film, which had predominantly featured young people, thus reinforcing the societal connection between young age, sexual agency, and 'sexiness'. Older people were no longer desexualised within film and television, and the shift to view older people in intimate and sexual relationships was, according to Vares (2009), located within the context of a broader (Western) cultural shift where sexual 'function' had come to be seen as a component of 'successful' ageing.

Through tracing the contours of sexual activity as a marker of successful ageing, Marshall (2010, 2011) described how this process was made possible by three key factors: (1) the arrival of the 'third age' cultural model of ageing; (2) the influence of demographic change on understandings of sexual health; and (3) the emphasis on preserving 'sexual fitness' as a central feature of the ageing-body project. The medicalisation of sexuality had already fashioned new standards of sexual performance, predominantly around heterosexual intercourse and sexual desire, for young women and men (Potts & Tiefer 2006). And sexuopharmaceuticals, like the erection-enhancing medicine Viagra, fitted this mould well. Both Gott (2005) and Marshall (2010) have described how the focus on fixing the sexual 'dysfunctions' associated with age, so that older people no longer needed to sexually retire, corresponded with the disease framework of ageing. The aim of sexuopharmaceuticals is to counter the impact of disease on sexual 'function', and we are currently in a position where "expectations of continued sexual functionality as an indicator of health in later life . . . underpin a growing medical and therapeutic industry" (Marshall 2011, p. 391). These messages are reflected in dominant public health discourses as leading institutions, including government bodies, promote the role of sexual activity to ageing health and well-being, including its ability to increase life-expectancy. While sexual activity and intimacy can have benefits to health and well-being, through connection with another person, physical exercise and the pleasure it gives us, the ability to increase our life expectancy is contested. New health agendas for older people have emerged with the message that to age well we should be sexually active. This counter-discourse – to the 'ageing as sexual decline' discourse – promotes the surveillance of sexual activity in older age, including the increasing medical attention that is paid to it (Marshall 2010).

Successful ageing, similar to the wider positive ageing movement, prescribes a form of governance where individuals are drawn, through regimes of health, into a personal responsibility for ageing well (Katz 2001). When older people's sexuality is considered within a neoliberalist framework, the responsibility lies on older people to *be* sexually active because to not do so would suggest they are not taking care of their health. One implication for those who cannot 'age well' in this way is a sense of failure and/or guilt. To 'age well' thus becomes a moral imperative. While the acknowledgement of the sexual health needs of older adults by institutions and authorities is a significant step forward, legitimating the area for further research and consequently the development of evidence-based recommendations for practice, there can be undesirable consequences when sexual activity is presented as essential to ageing well.

One of the tensions that arises when viewing the sexuality of older people through the lens of successful ageing therefore is that we need to ensure that in promoting the sexual rights of older people, in particular the right to be sexually active, we are not creating new (unrealistic and possibly undesired) expectations for older people. Indeed, one sexual right is the right *not* to be sexually active. A sexual rights framework for older people should be flexible so as to keep up with the dynamic field of sexualities, sexual health, and ageing. It should be adaptable to the diversity we find within this field, of which we learn more about as research progresses and marginalised voices are heard and responded to. A sexual rights framework for older people will provide individuals, family members, and health and social professionals a base from which to work. It will recognise that while people do not passively internalise the (ageist, sexist, homophobic, transphobic) messages of a society, these dominant messages have a cumulative effect (Nicolson 1993). In this way, they influence our self-perceptions and can render autonomy difficult to achieve.

Overview of this volume

All of the chapters that follow address the sexual rights of older people in different ways, from a range of disciplinary perspectives, and across heterosexual and non-binary gender and sexual identities. The authors draw attention to the cultural and social locations of older age and the ways that age can intersect with other social categories. By considering age-based inequality, they (naturally) turn to the impact of ageism upon older people's sexuality, including the resources available to them. The authors critique the research evidence and make recommendations for actions that need to be taken to overcome these issues. Key themes to emerge from the chapters as a whole include silencing, invisibility, prejudice, discrimination, and lack of awareness and understanding. None of the chapters deal specifically with law; however, we refer readers to Miller et al. (2015) for a discussion of the complexities of applying human rights law and policy to sexual rights, and, of course, the WHO report *Sexual Health, Human Rights and the Law* (2015).

We start with a description of sexual rights in Chapter 2, *Bundles of potential: the sexual rights of older people*, which 'sets the scene' for the whole collection and provides a sexual rights framework upon which the subsequent chapters draw. The proposed framework – an adaptation of the *World Association for Sexual Health* (WAS) sexual rights framework – covers 15 key domains, ranging from the right to privacy to the right to education.

In Chapter 3, *Framing the sexual rights of older heterosexual women: acknowledging diversity and change*, Rachel Thorpe, Bianca Fileborn, and Laura Hurd Clarke are mindful of the question: How can we rethink sexuality in later life in a way that does not negate older heterosexual women's sexual rights? Drawing on international research, they point out the diversity and fluidity of older women's experiences of sexual activity, and consider the tensions that arise when the 'sexy senior' sits along-side the 'asexual oldie'. They note that ageist and sexist discourses serve to neglect older women and have the potential to limit older women's sexual pleasure.

Similarly, in Chapter 4, *Older men's experiences of sexuality and their relevance for sexual rights*, Hans Wiggo Kristiansen and Linn J. Sandberg explore the ways that older heterosexual, gay, and bisexual men experience their sexuality. The authors highlight similarities and tensions among these groups to bring together an under-standing within a 'common framework' of ageing, masculinities, and subjectivities. Chapter 4 also notes that erection difficulties can impact a man's sense of self as masculine, but that men may renegotiate sex away from a phallocentric model. It, thus, shares with Chapter 10 attention to the dominant discourses of phallocentric sex, and the coital imperative, for sexual activity.

Both Chapters 3 and 4 highlight how powerful the social construction of gender and age can be in influencing ideas about the sexual desirability of older women and men. They reveal that narratives of successful ageing work to shape older women's and men's sexual subjectivities, but the 'ideal' presented may not 'match' older peo-ple's own self-perceptions, and consequently create a pressure to conform, or instil a sense of being different. Together, these chapters draw attention to the diversity of experiences of, and attitudes towards, later-life sexuality, and thus challenge the promotion of a 'one size fits all' approach to sexual rights.

In Chapter 5, *The hidden sexualities of older lesbians and bisexual women*, Sue West-wood and June Lowe discuss the intersections of ageism, sexism, and heterosexism to highlight the 'invisibilisation' of lesbians and bisexual women. Highlighting the varied sexualities of older women who are lesbian and bisexual, they argue that a lack of recognition of such diversity prevents women from being afforded sexual rights. They point out that the majority of stories about women's ageing relate to heterosexual women. Westwood and Lowe also argue that this 'sexually marginalised group' of older women, after a lifetime of living in secrecy, may be reluctant to disclose their identity to service providers and medical professionals as they wish to protect themselves from further discrimination: a situation that is exacerbated for older bisexual women given the current lack of understanding of bisexuality overall. They view invisibilisation as an ongoing process of exclusion and social marginalisation, and their suggestions to improve health and social care practice – to ensure inclusivity – include challenging the heteronormativity that already exists in services and increasing understanding of the issues that can affect older lesbians and bisexual women who may have 'reduced access to intergenerational support'.

Chapter 6 takes older transgender people as its focus and similarly notes the reduced support that comes from a lack of awareness and understanding. In *Transgender older people: at sea far from the sexual rights shore*, Loree Cook-Daniels and Michael Munson argue that asserting the sexual rights of older transgender people is not only a complicated process, but it is at times very difficult to attain. Again, discrimination and prejudice, often experienced over many years, can drive older transgender people to hide their gender identity in order to be safe. They often do not share their history with anyone, including health and social professionals, and delay or avoid accessing the services they need. Older transgender people can experience multiple barriers to getting help from appropriate services when they have been victims of violence. Sharing with Chapter 8, they do not fit the stereotype of the assault victim. Cook-Daniels and Munson note that the advent of the Internet has given transgender people a voice and a more widely recognised identity, something which has continued and developed into resources of support and community through the arrival of social media. However, they also warn that the sexual rights of older transgender people may not be high on the agenda of transgender organisations, which are still fighting for recognition of the basic human rights of transgender people.

In Chapter 7, *Intersex ageing and (sexual) rights*, J.R. Latham and M. Morgan Holmes acknowledge the absence of research and literature in the area, and because of this base their chapter around the experiences of two older intersex people and the film *Intersexion*. They argue that inhabiting an intersex body has made for a lifetime of contradiction, as bodies are hidden from 'prying eyes' due to a fear of social discrimination, while they are revealed, touched, and physically altered from childhood by medical professionals. Silence has traditionally surrounded the lives of those who are intersex; a silence that Latham and Holmes argue has perpetuated the abuse that intersex people can face. Being told they are different can enable feelings of shame to grow, and many intersex people have hidden their identity as a result. This makes children and young adults particularly vulnerable to abuse. But older intersex people can fear prejudice and discrimination that may come from their condition being revealed if they become dependent on others for care. Chapter 7 shares with Chapter 5 consideration of the ways that a lifetime of discrimination and violation of sexual rights can make older people fear for their health and social care: a fear that comes from being part of a marginalised group and from knowing that there is a lack of understanding among the general public, and health and social professionals.

Continuing the theme of silence and silencing, in Chapter 8, *Sexual assault of older women: breaking the silence*, Bianca Fileborn, Catherine Barrett, and Karen Roberto argue that the cultural constructions of gender and older age position women as fragile and powerless. The vulnerability of older women is exacerbated by the reality that those who report sexual assault may be dismissed on the basis that they do not 'fit' the stereotypical image of the female sexual assault victim, who is, quite simply, young. To not challenge this stereotype forms another violation of older people's sexual rights. Older women's experiences of sexual assault and the public and professional responses to those experiences are, thus, shaped by sexist and ageist forces. Similarly, understandings of what constitutes sexual assault are influenced by the 'cohort effect', in that older women in contemporary Western societies have lived most of their lives when rape within marriage was not legally recognised. Sharing with many of the chapters in this book, the authors highlight that the silencing of older sexual assault victims emanates from social prejudice and a lack of understanding.

In Chapter 9, *The challenges in reducing STIs while fulfilling and enhancing the sexual rights of older people*, Graham Brown, Anthony Lyons, Sharron Hinchliff, and Pauline Crameri tackle the ever-increasing diagnoses of sexually transmitted infections (STIs) in the older age groups. The authors examine the evidence and developments in responding to STIs among older people and the associated challenges in reducing STIs while being sure to fulfil their sexual rights. They argue that older people have been neglected within safer-sex campaigns as a result of ageist beliefs, including the assumption that they are not sexually active, or if they are they do not take sexual risks. Again, the social construction of old age has limited awareness and understanding of sexual behaviours, and consequently the resources and strategies that promote sexual health in these older cohorts. Suggested implications for practice and health promotion campaigns include making sure that they are tailored specifically to older people and not making the assumption that the tools and strategies that work with younger people will also be successful with their older counterparts.

Catherine Barrett, Emily Wentzell, and Rafaella Ferrero Camoletto explore the 'viagrization of male sexuality' and its implications for understanding erectile dysfunction (ED) in Chapter 10, *Challenging the 'viagrization' of heterosexuality and ageing*. The authors argue that this medical technology, which became a 'treatment' for ED in the mid-1990s, has redefined male sexual problems while promoting wider awareness of ED. Challenging the phallocentric model of sex and ageist discourses, they critique the view that the sexual rights of older people equate with the 'right to access medical intervention to continue youthful and normative forms of sexuality'. They provide an alternative position: sex-positive approaches through accessible education that support (diverse) sexual expression in later life. The relational context of Viagra use is highlighted, with the important but often neglected point that Viagra may not be in the best interests of men and/or their female partners (the chapter takes a heterosexual focus because of the limited evidence on Viagra use among older men who have sex with men), and that older men often renegotiate intimacy away from a model of sex that requires an erect penis (see also Chapter 4). Indeed, even the 'sex specialists' who are quoted in this chapter question the way that Viagra has influenced men's sexual rights, pointing out the consumerism attached to the 'hyperreal notion of ageless sexuality'.

The penultimate chapter, *Older people as cyber-sexual beings: online and Internet dating* (Chapter 11), by Sue Malta and Summer Roberts, addresses the increasing use of Internet dating sites by older people who wish to meet sexual and romantic partners. New websites aimed specifically at this cohort are increasing; however, existing websites, previously aimed only at young people, have been found to engage in age-related discrimination by placing higher charges for older clients to use their services. Internet dating brings both opportunities and risks for older people, for example, the chance to 'explore and enhance their sexual expression' in a society that often denies them this right, to dangers to their sexual health, sexual well-being, and personal safety when meeting face-to-face with a partner who they first met online. The authors conclude that in order to ensure that sexual rights are being met, safety measures need to be put in place to address the risks to older users as well as younger ones. The latter currently receive the bulk of information and sexual health education about the use of dating websites.

In the final chapter (Chapter 12), *Conclusion: moving forward, implementing change*, we draw together the key points and recommendations from the previous chapters to address the challenges that come from asserting the sexual rights of older people. We describe strategies for raising awareness of these rights, including critical sexuality studies, to build evidence around rights violations and to engage communities in debating and constructing strategies for reform. We suggest that education and awareness-raising can be a first step in helping to improve understanding of the sexual rights of older people, among older people themselves, and those whose work brings them into contact with older people. We end by making recommendations for future directions in professional practice and service delivery, policy making, and research.

Notes

1 According to the World Health Organization, life expectancy in South Africa for women and men is low (see: www.who.int/countries/zaf/en/), which may explain the definition of older that was used in this study.
2 A 'general practitioner' works in a similar capacity to a 'family physician', and both terms refer to doctors who work in a primary care setting.

References

Barbre, JW 1998, 'Meno-boomers and moral guardians: An exploration of the cultural construction of menopause', in R Weitz (ed.), *The politics of women's bodies: Sexuality, appearance and behaviour*, Oxford University Press, Oxford.

Calasanti, TM & Slevin, KF 2006, 'Introduction: Age matters', in TM Calasanti & KF Slevin (eds.), *Age matters: Realigning feminist thinking*, Routledge, New York.

Department of Health 2013, *A framework for sexual health improvement in England*, HMSO, London.

Gott, M 2005, *Sexuality, sexual health and ageing*, Open University Press, England.

Gott, M & Hinchliff, S 2003, 'How important is sex in later life? The views of older people', *Social Science & Medicine*, vol. 56, pp. 1617–1628.

Gott, M, Hinchliff, S & Galena, E 2004, 'General practitioner attitudes to discussing sexual health issues with older people', *Social Science & Medicine*, vol. 58, pp. 2093–2103.

Hawkes, G 1996, *A sociology of sex and sexuality*, Open University Press, England.

Heidari, S 2015, 'Sexual rights and bodily integrity as human rights', *Reproductive Health Matters*, vol. 23, no. 46, pp. 1–6.

Hinchliff, S & Gott, M 2011, 'Seeking medical help for sexual concerns in mid and later life: A review of the literature', *Annual Review of Sex Research*, vol. 48, no. 2, pp. 106–111.

Kaighobadi, F, Konx, J, Reddy, V & Sandfort, T 2014, 'Age and sexual risk among black men who have sex with men in South Africa: The mediating role of attitudes towards condoms', *Journal of Health Psychology*, vol. 19, no. 10, pp. 1271–1278.

Karlsson, SG & Borrell, K 2005, 'A home of their own: Women's boundary work in LAT relationships', *Journal of Aging Studies*, vol. 19, pp. 73–84.

Katz, S 2001, 'Growing older without aging? Positive aging, antiageism, and anti-aging', *Generations*, vol. 25, no. 4, pp. 27–32.

Lenoir, MA & Dortch, L 2011, 'Sexual rights: A new paradigm in addressing Sexual and Reproductive Health (SRH) in sexual health: A public health challenge in Europe', *Entre Nous*, no. 72, viewed 11 August 2015, www.euro.who.int/en/health-topics/ Life-stages/sexual-and-reproductive-health/publications/entre-nous/entre-nous/ sexual-health-a-public-health-challenge-in-europe.-entre-nous-72,-2011

Macdowall, W, Gibson, LJ, Tanton, C, Mercer, CH, Lewis, R, Clifton, S, Field, N, Datta, J, Sonnenberg, P, Erens, B, Copas, AJ, Phelps, A, Prah, P, Jonson, AM & Wellings, K 2013, 'Lifetime prevalence, associated factors, and circumstances of non-volitional sex in women and men in Britain: Findings from the third National Survey of Sexual Attitudes and Lifestyles (Natsal-3)', *Lancet*, vol. 382, no. 9907, pp. 1845–1855, viewed 27 September 2015, www.ncbi.nlm.nih.gov/pmc/articles/PMC3898964/

Marshall, BL 2010, 'Science, medicine and virility surveillance: "Sexy seniors" in the pharmaceutical imagination', *Sociology of Health & Illness*, vol. 32, no. 2, pp. 211–224.

Marshall, BL 2011, 'The graying of "sexual health": A critical research agenda', *Canadian Review of Sociology/Revue canadienne de sociologie*, vol. 48, no. 4, pp. 390–413.

Marshall, BL & Katz, S 2006, 'From androgyny to androgens: Resexing the aging body', in TM Calasanti & KF Slevin (eds.), *Age matters: Realigning feminist thinking*, Routledge, New York.

Miller, AM, Kismödi, E, Cottingham, J & Gruskin, S 2015, 'Sexual rights as human rights: A guide to authoritative sources and principles for applying human rights to sexuality and sexual health', *Reproductive Health Matters*, vol. 23, no. 46, pp. 16–30.

Minichiello, V, Browne, J & Kendig, H 2000, 'Perceptions and consequences of ageism: Views of older people', *Ageing & Society*, vol. 20, no. 3, pp. 253–278.

Nicolson, P 1993, 'Public values and private beliefs: Why do women refer themselves for sex therapy?', in JM Ussher & CD Baker (eds.), *Psychological perspectives on sexual problems: New directions for theory and practice*, Routledge, London.

Park, A, Curtice, J, Thomson, K, Phillips, M, Johnson, M & Clery, E 2008, *British social attitudes: The 24th report*, Sage, London.

Potts, A & Tiefer, L 2006, 'Introduction', *Sexualities*, vol. 9, p. 267.

Reuben, DR 1970, *Everything you ever wanted to know about sex*, W.H. Allen, London.

Tiefer, L 1995, *Sex is not a natural act and other essays*, Westview Press, Boulder, CO.

Vares, T 2009, 'Reading the "sexy oldie": Gender, age(ing) and embodiment', *Sexualities*, vol. 12, no. 4, pp. 503–524.

Williams, A, Ylänne, V, Wadleigh, PM, Williams, A, Ylänne, V & Wadleigh, PM 2007, Selling the "elixir of life": Images of the elderly in an Olivio advertising campaign. *Journal of Aging Studies*, vol. 21, pp. 1–21.

World Health Organization 2006, *Defining sexual health: Report of a technical consultation on sexual health 28–31 January 2002, Geneva*, World Health Organization, viewed 18 March 2017 www.who.int/reproductivehealth/publications/sexual_health/defining_sexual_health.pdf

World Health Organization 2015, *Sexual health, human rights and the law*, World Health Organization, viewed 20 December 2016, http://apps.who.int/iris/handle/10665/175556

World Health Organization 2016, *Global health observatory: Life expectancy*, World Health Organization, viewed 29 December 2016, www.who.int/gho/mortality_burden_disease/life_tables/situation_trends/en/

2

BUNDLES OF POTENTIAL

The sexual rights of older people

Catherine Barrett and Sharron Hinchliff

Introduction

In the previous chapter we described the importance of understanding older people's sexuality. In this chapter we outline a sexual rights framework for older people. We begin by exploring what we mean by rights, or the potential of every person and the entitlement to thrive. We then explore the development of an international declaration of sexual rights by the World Association of Sexual Health and consider the application of these rights to the lives and potential of older people.

We finish with a critique of the rights-based approach and suggest how the limitations of and obstacles to a sexual rights-based approach can be addressed in a framework for the sexual rights of older people. We conclude by reflecting on the opportunities presented by our Declaration of the Sexual Rights of Older People and suggest there is an opportunity for new discourses about what can reasonably be done to maximize older people's potential in a broad range of cultural contexts.

A bundle of human potential: the significance of rights

Human rights are described by Plummer (2013) as distinctive and unique potentials or capabilities for life that are shaped and facilitated by the social aspects of our lives. Plummer (2010) draws on the work of feminist philosopher Martha Nussbaum to suggest these capabilities include emotions; practical reason; affiliation; play; control over one's environment; bodily integrity; sexual satisfaction; and freedom from sexual violence. Plummer evocatively suggests that humans are bundles of potential and capabilities that need the appropriate social conditions in order to flourish (Plummer, 2001). These social conditions include human rights (Plummer, 2010) that clarify the equal worth of people (Plummer, 2001).

The spotlight on human rights and potential is increasingly focused on older people. This shift can be traced to 1982 when an International Plan of Action on Ageing adopted by the World Assembly articulated that the respect for and authority of older people in traditional societies was under threat (United Nations, 1983). A review of the Plan in 2002 committed to the full realization of all human rights and freedoms of older people (United Nations, 2002). A decade later, for the first time, a Report of the Secretary-General to the General Assembly of the United Nations focused on the human rights of older persons and noted the lack of participation in policy making and political life (United Nations, 2011). Then, in 2012, the UN General Assembly established an Open-Ended Working Group on strengthening the protection of the human rights of older persons.

Despite these shifts, older people are still not recognised explicitly under international human rights laws, leading to growing calls for a convention on the rights of older people (HelpAge International, undated). Older people's human rights continue to fall short across the globe, so perhaps it is not surprising that their sexual rights are also lagging. It is in this context that we propose a framework of sexual rights of older people – to ensure sexuality is considered fundamental to recognizing the human potential of older people.

The invention of sexual rights

The World Association for Sexual Health (WAS) developed a declaration of sexual rights in 1999. They evolved to focus on the issues of family planning and violence against women, and then later the fight against discrimination based on sexual orientation and gender identities (Giami, 2015).

The Declaration gives pre-eminence to sexual rights and places sexual health and the recognition of the benefits of sexual pleasure on general health at the heart of the debate. It makes connections with human rights, particularly the fight against violence and discrimination and the promotion of civil liberties (World Association for Sexual Health, 1999). It emphasizes the empowerment of individuals and examines sexual health concerns within a human rights framework, with the goals to promote awareness and advocacy of sexual issues and especially to facilitate better education and sexual health services (Lottes and Adkins, 2003)

The Declaration moved quickly around the world, with many countries developing their own programs to promote sexual rights (Plummer, 2001), but there have also been critiques of the sexual rights approach, with some countries and religions having no place for them (Plummer, 2010).

Despite the broad take-up of the Declaration, there has been little recognition of its application to older people. There is an ever-growing field of scientific inquiry around older people's sexuality, but almost nothing has been done to explore or address the sexual rights of older people (Aboderin, 2014). There is evidence that older people experience sexual inequalities, but little has been documented about the nature of their sexual rights and the key barriers they face to accessing services (Aboderin, 2014).

To address the gap in recognition of older people's sexual rights, this chapter takes the WAS Declaration of Sexual Rights and applies it to the lives of older people. Fifteen of the 16 sexual rights were found to relate to older people, and only one, a right on decisions relating to childbirth, has not been utilised. In Table 2.1, a summary statement for each of the 15 Rights is presented. Each right has been adapted to explicitly refer to older people and aspects of their lives.

TABLE 2.1 Declaration of the Sexual Rights of Older People

1. **The right to equality and non-discrimination**

   Older people have the right to enjoy all the sexual rights set out in this declaration without distinction of any kind, particularly related to age.

2. **The right to life, liberty and security**

   Older people have the right to life, liberty and security that cannot be arbitrarily threatened, limited or taken away for reasons related to sexuality.

3. **The right to autonomy and bodily integrity**

   Older people have the right to control and decide freely on matters related to their sexuality and their body. This includes the choices of sexual behaviours, practices, partners and relationships with due regard to the rights of others.

4. **The right to be free from torture and cruel, inhuman or degrading treatment or punishment**

   Older people have the right to be free from torture and cruel, inhuman or degrading treatment or punishment related to sexuality.

5. **The right to be free from all forms of violence and coercion**

   Older people have the right to be free from sexuality related violence and coercion.

6. **The right to privacy**

   Older people have the right to privacy related to sexuality, sexual life and choices regarding their own body and consensual sexual relations and practices without arbitrary interferences and intrusion.

7. **The right to the highest attainable standard of health including sexual health**

   Older people have the right to the highest attainable level of health and wellbeing in relation to sexuality, including the possibility of pleasurable, satisfying and safe sexual experiences.

8. **The right to enjoy the benefits of scientific progress and its application**

   Older people have the right to enjoy the benefits of scientific progress and its applications in relation to sexuality and ageing and sexual health.

9. **The right to information**

   Older people have the right to access scientifically accurate and understandable information related to sexuality and ageing, sexual health and sexual rights through diverse sources.

10. **The right to education and the right to comprehensive sexuality education**

    Older people have the right to education and comprehensive sexuality education that is age appropriate and grounded in a positive approach to sexuality, ageing and older people.

(Continued)

TABLE 2.1 (Continued)

---

11. **The right to enter, form and dissolve marriage and other similar types of relationships**

    Older people have the right to choose whether or not to marry and to enter freely and with full and free consent into marriage, partnership or other similar relationships.

12. **The right to freedom of thought, opinion and expression**

    Older people have the right to freedom of thought, opinion and expression regarding sexuality and the right to express their own sexuality with due respect to the rights of others.

13. **The right to freedom of association and peaceful assembly**

    Older people have the right to peacefully organise, associate, assemble, demonstrate and advocate including about sexuality, sexual health and sexual rights.

14. **The right to participation in public and political life**

    Older people are entitled to an environment that enables active, free and meaningful participation in and contribution to the civil, economic, social, political, and other aspects of human life.

15. **The right to access justice, remedies and redress**

    Older people have the right to access justice, remedies and redress for violations of their sexual rights.

Rights in practice: what these mean to older people

In this section we describe how the sexual rights of older people may be experienced. We begin by providing a statement of each right in full and exploring the barriers and enablers to enactment of each right. Then we outline reforms required to ensure that older people's sexual rights are achieved.

Equality and non-discrimination (#1)

> *Older people are entitled to enjoy all sexual rights set out in this declaration without distinction of any kind, such as race, ethnicity, color, gender, sex, language, religion, political or other opinion, national or social origin, place of residence, property, birth, disability, age, nationality, marital or family status, sexual orientation, gender identity and expression, health status, economic and social situation and other status.*

The first right in the Declaration explicitly refers to sexual rights without distinction related to age and notes that this forms the foundation for the remaining sexual rights. This acknowledgement that ageism is an obstacle to sexual rights is particularly pertinent to older people. As described in the previous chapter, in Western cultures ageing is conceptualized as decline (Gullette, 2015), resulting in perceptions of older people as asexual and a failure to recognize or address sexual rights. Ageism can also result in older people internalizing messages of decline and asexuality. This in turn can erode older people's sense of self-worth, identity and wellbeing (George, 1998) and result in older people believing that sexual wellbeing is not something they can reasonably expect (Barrett, 2011).

These ageist beliefs need to be challenged in order to ensure that old age is not a barrier to achieving sexual rights. It is also important to consider gender in this context. Reforms to address gender inequality are relatively recent, and older women may experience gender inequalities relating to their sexual rights. This is particularly obvious in the chapters on sexual assault (Chapter 8) and Viagra (Chapter 10).

Life, liberty and security (#2)

> Older people have the right to life, liberty and security that cannot be arbitrarily threatened, limited or taken away for reasons related to sexuality. These include sexual orientation, consensual sexual behaviour and practices, gender identity and expression or because of accessing or providing services related to sexual and reproductive health.

Perhaps the clearest examples of restrictions to older people's life and security relates to the lives of older lesbian, gay, bisexual, trans and intersex (LGBTI) people. In many countries being LGBT is still a crime punishable by death. Additionally, older intersex people may encounter threats to their liberty and security (Latham and Barrett, 2015a). Older LGBTI people may feel the need to hide their sexual orientation, gender identity or sex because of the fear of violence and abuse or the loss of employment, family and friends (Crameri et al., 2015). Disclosure may also result in discrimination in health and aged care services (Barrett, 2009).

More broadly speaking, older people who express their sexuality may also find their liberties restricted by family members or service providers who believe older people should be asexual and sexual expression should be repressed (Barrett, 2011). The use of medications or other actions to suppress libido is likely to be significantly reduced if a sexual rights-based lens is applied.

Autonomy and bodily integrity (#3)

> Older people have the right to control and decide freely on matters related to their sexuality and their body. This includes the choices of sexual behaviours, practices, partners and relationships with due regard to the rights of others. Free and informed decision-making requires free and informed consent prior to any sexually related testing, interventions, therapies, surgeries or research.

Autonomy is so important in the lives of older people that the World Health Organization's Framework for Active Ageing (2002) has at its heart a goal to maintain autonomy and independence. This approach challenges the commonly held view that all older people lose the capacity to make informed decisions, particularly in relation to sexuality. Older people who express their sexuality may be judged as incompetent because of the decision they have made – rather than their cognitive status.

Autonomy may also be challenged by adults whose parents undertake gender transition or form a same-sex relationship later in life (Barrett et al., 2015). These decisions may also be questioned by staff in residential aged care who report concerns about offending other residents (Barrett, 2011). The lack of respect for older people's right to decide in these situations results in their sexual right to make decisions about sexual behaviours, practices and relationships not being respected.

Degrading treatment or punishment (#4)

Older people have the right to be free from torture and cruel, inhuman or degrading treatment or punishment related to sexuality including that which is perpetrated for reasons related to someone's sex, gender, sexual orientation, gender identity and expression and bodily diversity.

Degrading treatment or punishment may be perpetrated against older people in response to expression of sexuality, sex or gender. This can range from ageist mocking of older people, to the use of chemical restraints or withdrawal of family support or services (Barrett, Harrison and Kent 2009). Older LGBTI people may be particularly vulnerable to vilification in the workplace or community. They may also have services refused or withdrawn if their sexual orientation, gender identity or sex is revealed (Latham and Barrett, 2015b; Barrett et al., 2015).

The degrading treatment or punishment experienced by older people who express their sexuality, and particularly by older LGBTI people, highlights the importance of recognizing that sexuality is a rights-based issue for older people.

Violence and coercion (#5)

Everyone shall be free from sexuality related violence and coercion, including rape, sexual abuse, sexual harassment bullying, sexual exploitation, and violence committed because of real or perceived sexual practices, sexual orientation, gender identity and expression and bodily diversity.

The issue of the sexuality related violence experienced by older people, particularly older women, is being thrown into focus with the growing recognition of the problem of family violence and elder abuse. Older women experience sexual assault in their own homes, in institutional settings and in public places, and these assaults are perpetrated by intimate partners, family members, service providers and strangers (Mann et al., 2014). Underpinning the lack of action to prevent the sexual assault of older women is the myth that old age is a protective factor against sexual assault – in other words, the belief that older women do not experience sexual assault because they are not sexually attractive (Mann et al., 2014).

A further obstacle to the lack of recognition of older women's right to be free from sexual violence is the cultural effect of marital rape laws. In some countries, rape in marriage is interpreted as the state-sanctioned right of a man's access to a woman's body on the grounds of his rights to sexual fulfilment within marriage (Richardson, 2000).

Societal attitudes contribute to the vulnerability of women to sexual violence and coercion (Hollomotz, 2009), and combined with ageism they act as a significant barrier to older women achieving this right. Older women who pick up these messages that there is not permission to report sexual assault are less likely to report assault when it occurs (Mann et al., 2014). There is a need to address the sexual assault of older women in strategies to prevent violence against women and in strategies to prevent elder abuse – to recognize older women's right to be free from sexual violence and coercion.

Privacy (#6)

Older people have the right to privacy related to sexuality, sexual life and choices regarding their own body and consensual sexual relations and practices without arbitrary interferences and intrusion. This includes the right to control the disclosure of sexuality related personal information to others.

Privacy is a fundamental human right and has become one of the most important human rights issues of the modern age. It is also a right that may be significantly compromised for older people who are reliant on family members and service providers for care or support. This dependency on others can mean that sexual expression and choices that were once private, become public. As a consequence, older people's decisions may be overridden and personal information shared with family members, by service providers who are concerned that sexual choices are always bad choices (Barrett, 2011).

Privacy is also a considerable issue for older LGBTI people. The increased interest in LGBTI inclusive aged care services may result in older LGBTI people being asked to disclose their sexual orientation, gender identity and intersex status. While this may be viewed by service providers as an important step in LGBTI inclusivity, it can be experienced by older LGBTI people as an invasion of privacy and generate considerable concern in those who have historical experiences of discrimination in health services. Service providers need to understand the privacy implications of LGBTI inclusive assessment and inform older LGBTI people how this information will be used, stored and with whom it will be shared (Crameri et al., 2015).

Health, pleasurable and safe sexual experiences (#7)

Older people have the right to the highest attainable level of health and wellbeing in relation to sexuality, including the possibility of pleasurable, satisfying and safe sexual experiences. This requires the availability, accessibility, acceptability of quality health services and access to the conditions that influence and determine health including sexual health.

To achieve the highest attainable level of health and wellbeing in relation to sexuality, older people need information about their sexual health and wellbeing. The chapters in this edited volume highlight that there is little evidence this has occurred. For example, Chapters 8, 9 and 11 describe the lack of information provided to older people to prevent sexual assault and promote safe sexual experiences and Chapter 10 explores the lack of information to support older men coping with age-related erectile decline.

It is likely that change to address this gap will begin by prioritizing rights violations such as the sexual assault of older women or aspects of sexuality where there are clear 'medical problems'. It is also important that change encompasses all the rights outlined in this Declaration, including the right to pleasure and satisfying sexual experiences.

Scientific progress and its application (#8)

> *Older people have the right to enjoy the benefits of scientific progress and its applications in relation to sexuality and sexual health.*

The benefits, and complexities, of scientific progress on older people's sexuality are exemplified in the use of sexuopharmaceuticals by older men (see Chapter 10). Progress in this area has been driven by pharmaceutical companies – and highlights the void in addressing the sexual rights of older people. The trends of anti-ageing medicine and the cultural narrative of 'successful ageing' position ageing as undesirable and place responsibility on older people to actively resist growing old through technology use (Joyce et al., 2015). The uptake of sexuopharmaceuticals is spurred by our failure to address other sexual rights – including the right to information on age-related erectile decline and the right to comprehensive sexuality education that takes a positive approach to sexuality.

As scientific progress continues, it will continue to accentuate our lack of attention to societal and cultural attitudes, which underpin much of the sexual rights.

Information provision (#9)

> *Older people have the right to access scientifically accurate and understandable information related to sexuality, sexual health and sexual rights through diverse sources. Such information should not be arbitrarily censored, withheld or intentionally misrepresented.*

The provision of information to older people on their sexual rights is incredibly important. The availability of information to older people is one of the World Health Organisation's (2015) measures of age-friendly communities. They note that information is essential for informed decision making and should be provided in a way that is inclusive of people across a range of age groups and functional abilities, who may vary in their preferred mode of communication. Information for older people also needs to take into account opportunities for lifelong learning and help older people develop the skills and confidence they need to adapt and stay independent (World Health Organisation, 2002), particularly in relation to their sexuality.

There is little evidence that information on sexuality is developed for older people, and this is a key factor in cultural change to achieve their sexual rights.

Comprehensive sexuality education (#10)

Older people have the right to education and comprehensive sexuality education. Comprehensive sexuality education must be age appropriate, scientifically accurate, culturally competent and grounded in human rights, gender equality and a positive approach to sexuality, ageing and pleasure.

Few, if any, countries provide comprehensive sexuality education for older people, and yet doing so could be a powerful tool in promoting older people's sexual rights. Older people could be supported to critique existing discourses about sexuality and ageing, particularly those in the West that medicalise the ageing body and sexuality (Lamb, 2015) and those that place the responsibility on older people to fight their ageing and present themselves as ageless and sexy (Marshall, 2015). Older people could be encouraged to develop a strong, embodied sense of their sexual selves and who they want to be. Education could take into account the physical and psychosocial factors that impact on sexual health as well as the impacts of increasing age and disability (Barrett, 2011).

Educational approaches need to recognize that these adult learners are capable and are likely to want to be involved in planning their learning (Knowles, 1973). Older people could be supported as peer educators to ensure that education is age appropriate and culturally competent. Peer educators are credible and influential role models who could empower others (Turner and Shepherd, 1999). Peer education has been used in other contexts to improve health outcomes for older people (Cattan et al., 2005; Rose, 1992), and older peer educators have been reported to be effective role models, reach marginalized groups and influence changes in behavior (Peel and Warburton, 2009).

Relationships (#11)

Older people have the right to choose whether or not to marry and to enter freely and with full and free consent into marriage, partnership or other similar relationships. All persons are entitled to equal rights entering into, during, at a dissolution or marriage, partnership or other similar relationship, without discrimination of exclusion of any kind. This right includes equal entitlements to social welfare and other benefits regardless of the form of relationships.

As divorce rates increase and older people live longer, there are more opportunities for older people to renegotiate their sexuality and form new relationships in later life. While new relationships have much to offer in terms of intimacy and sex, they can also be a significant source of family conflict. Older heterosexuals who form new relationships may find their decisions are not supported by their children, who are grieving the loss of their parents' relationships or their loss of status and inheritance.

Similarly, older LGB people who form same-sex relationships later in life may find adult children from their previous heterosexual relationship do not approve of their new same-sex identity and actively subvert their right to make informed choices about relationships and sexuality (Barrett et al., 2015).

The entitlement to enter into a new relationship may also be questioned for older people who live in residential aged care facilities. Perceptions of asexuality may result in questioning a resident's capacity to make an informed choice about a relationship. In such cases, Everett (2007) notes that intervening should only occur if the risk is unreasonable and the resident is incapable or if harm is being done to others. This risk needs to be differentiated from attempts to eradicate sexual expression in response to the discomfort of staff, family members or other residents.

Freedom of thought, opinion and expression (#12)

> *Older people have the right to freedom of thought, opinion and expression regarding sexuality and the right to express their own sexuality through, for example, appearance, communication and behaviour with due respect to the rights of others.*

Older people who express their sexuality may encounter ridicule in the broader community. Their loss of autonomy or dependence on family members may mean expressions of intimacy (hugging, kissing, touching) or sexual pleasure (intercourse, masturbation) may be blocked by family members or service providers who feel older people should not be sexual.

This may also be the case for trans people, with family members placing restrictions on gender appearance (Barrett et al., 2015) or service providers determining how a resident is allowed to present themselves in residential aged care (Latham and Barrett, 2015b).

It is important that sexual expression is viewed as a right that older people have, and this needs to be addressed in community education campaigns as well as information provided to health practitioners. There is also a need to provide older people with the information on how to assert their rights.

Freedom of association and peaceful assembly (#13)

> *Older people have the right to peacefully organize, associate, assemble, demonstrate and advocate, including about sexuality, sexual health and sexual rights.*

The right to freedom of association and to advocate are particularly pertinent to the lives of older LGBTI people. While the violations of LGBTI people's rights are recognized in many countries around the world – there has been limited focus on older LGBTI community members. Older LGBTI people have the right to connect, to speak out and to form communities. More broadly speaking, there are few examples of older people speaking out about their rights. However, if we provide more spaces for older people to participate in public and political life, this may occur.

Participation in public and political life (#14)

> Older people are entitled to an environment that enables active, free and meaningful partici-
> pation in and contribution to the civil, economic, social, political, and other aspects of human
> life at local, national, regional and international levels. In particular, older people are entitled
> to participate in the development and implementation of policies that determine their welfare,
> including their sexuality and sexual health, and that influence the design of health and aged
> care services.

The World Health Organisation (2002) notes that central to a human rights-based
approach is the importance of ensuring that older people participate actively and
make informed decisions about their health and wellbeing. In their framework
for Active Ageing, they add that optimizing participation is a core process that
can improve ageing and health and promote accountability by empowering older
people to claim their rights.

Opportunities have been missed to engage older people in contributing to the
development of policy, education and services that promote their sexual health and
wellbeing. Older people are a great source of wisdom and information, and the
engagement of older people in shaping sexuality policies could help ensure the
effectiveness of such policies.

Justice, remedies and redress (#15)

> Older people have the right to access justices, remedies and redress for violations of their sexual
> rights. This requires effective, adequate, accessible and appropriate educative, legislative, judicial
> and other measures. Remedies include redress through restitution, compensation, rehabilitation,
> satisfaction and guarantee of non-repetition.

The lack of recognition of older people's sexual rights results in few opportunities
for justice, remedies and redress when these rights are violated. This status quo is
also perpetuated by older people who have internalized the ageist views of their
communities and may not feel a sense of entitlement to accessing advocacy or support services. This is particularly apparent in the context of the sexual assault of
older women, wherein older women who report sexual assault are unlikely to be
heard or believed, and therefore justice is unlikely (Mann et al., 2014).

The sexual rights of older people need to be recognized and enacted, and there
needs to be justice and redress when rights are violated. Without avenues for justice
and redress, the motivation to recognize rights is restricted.

Barriers and limitations of a rights-based approach

These sexual rights of older people could provide a useful framework for government bodies, policy-makers, researchers, service providers, educators and older
people themselves. They could enable new conversations to take place, new questions to be asked and new approaches to be considered. They are not intended as

a mandate, but we acknowledge that sexual rights have limitations and encounter barriers.

Perhaps one of the most significant critiques about the International Declaration of Sexual Rights relates to cultural relativism. It has been argued that sexual rights are simply a Western concept of limited value and that the behaviours and customs of a society should be evaluated within the context of its own culture and not with respect to outside universal standards (Lottes, 2013). Communities may have competing and conflicting goals, and individual sexual rights cannot be viewed as separate from their cultural context (Plummer, 2012).

And then within countries and communities, conflict and inequalities also exist and may be significant barriers to the sexual rights of older people. Conflict arises in relation to sexuality, which has become a touchstone for fear, predjudice and hatred (Altman and Beyer, 2014). For example, religious organisations, like The Holy See, are a staunch opponent of a sexual rights agenda (Beattie, 2014; Coates et al., 2014).

Inequalities also exist in relation to social context (Wellings et al., 2006). Sexuality cannot be understood apart from social, political and economic structures or without reference to the cultural discourses that give sexuality meaning (Parker, 2007). It is difficult to talk about sexual rights without addressing equalities in the distribution of power, money and resources (Cottingham et al., 2010). In wealthier countries, personal choice is greater than in poorer countries (Wellings et al., 2006); income and education influence the choices that individuals can make (Ory et al., 2003); and for those who do not have fundamental human rights, sexual rights are a luxury (Plummer, 2005).

Inequalities also exist in relation to gender. The lack of attention to the social worlds of older people's sexuality also fails to acknowledge the influence of gender, particularly power differentials and men's privilege. We have added gender to the first standard in recognition of this fact. We also suggest that cultural, social, economic and religious context provides important information for understanding how these rights can be applied. Indeed, this information must be taken into account in the developing of local responses to the sexual rights of older people.

Discussion

Taking into account these limitations, it is important to reflect on the role of sexual rights. The sexual rights outlined in this chapter seek to raise the standard, rather than provide a prescription to be applied to all contexts. They have discursive power and influence on legislation (Foley, 2012). These sexual rights of older people offer a new opportunity for communication and dialogue. Rights can only exist in dialogue with others (Plummer, 2001). This is a dialogue we need to have. It is important to ask: What sexual rights do older people have? How are they enacted?

Throughout our lives, we accumulate sexual beliefs about who we are and what is expected of us (Simon and Gagnon, 2011). This raises questions about what messages we send to older people about who they are and what is expected of them. There is unlikely to be international consensus on the sexual rights of older people. There isn't consensus on human rights more broadly speaking (Sheill, 2006), but that is not the point. The point is that the rights give us a new starting point for conversation about what currently is and what we want it to be.

References

Aboderin, I., 2014. Sexual and reproductive health and rights of older men and women: Addressing a policy blind spot. *Reproductive Health Matters*, *22*(44), pp. 185–190.

Altman, D. and Beyrer, C., 2014. The global battle for sexual rights. *Journal of the International AIDS Society*, *17*(1).

Barrett, C.M., 2011. Auditing organisational capacity to promote the sexual health of older people. *Electronic Journal of Applied Psychology*, *7*(1), pp. 31–36.

Barrett, C.M., 2008. *My people: A project exploring the experiences of gay, lesbian, bisexual, transgender and intersex seniors in aged-care services.* Melbourne, Matrix Guild Victoria Incorporated.

Barrett, C.M., Crameri, P., Lambourne, S., Latham, J.R. and Whyte, C., 2015. Understanding the experiences and needs of lesbian, gay, bisexual and trans Australians living with dementia, and their partners. *Australasian Journal on Ageing*, *34*(S2), pp. 34–38.

Barrett, C.M., Harrison, J. and Kent, J., 2009. *Permission to speak: Determining strategies towards the development of gay, lesbian, bisexual, transgender and intersex friendly aged care services in Victoria.* Melbourne, Matrix Guild of Victoria Incorporated.

Beattie, T., 2014. Whose rights, which rights? The United Nations, the Vatican, gender and sexual and reproductive rights. *The Heythrop Journal*, *55*(6), pp. 1080–1090.

Cattan, M., White, M., Bond, J. and Learmouth, A., 2005. Preventing social isolation and loneliness among older people: A systematic review of health promotion interventions. *Ageing and Society*, *25*(1), pp. 41–67.

Coates, A.L., Hill, P.S., Rushton, S. and Balen, J., 2014. The Holy See on sexual and reproductive health rights: Conservative in position, dynamic in response. *Reproductive Health Matters*, *22*(44), pp. 114–124.

Cottingham, J., Kismodi, E., Hilber, A.M., Lincetto, O., Stahlhofer, M. and Gruskin, S., 2010. Using human rights for sexual and reproductive health: Improving legal and regulatory frameworks. *Bulletin of the World Health Organization*, *88*(7), pp. 551–555.

Crameri, P., Barrett, C., Latham, J.R. and Whyte, C., 2015. It is more than sex and clothes: Culturally safe services for older lesbian, gay, bisexual, transgender and intersex people. *Australasian Journal on Ageing*, *34*(S2), pp. 21–25.

Everett, B., 2007. Ethically managing sexual activity in long-term care. *Sexuality and Disability*, *25*(1), pp. 21–27.

Foley, S., 2012. The UN convention on the rights of persons with disabilities: A paradigm shift in the sexual empowerment of adults with down syndrome or more sound and fury signifying nothing? *Sexuality and Disability*, *30*(4), pp. 381–393.

George, L.K., 1998. Self and identity in later life: Protecting and enhancing the self. *Journal of Aging and Identity*, *3*(3), pp. 133–152.

Giami, A., 2015. Sexuality, health and human rights: The invention of sexual rights. *Sexologies*, *24*(3), pp. e45–e53.

Gullette, M.M., 2015. Aged by culture. In J. Twigg and W. Martin (eds.), *Routledge handbook of cultural gerontology*, pp. 21–28. London, Routledge.

HelpAge International, undated. Strengthening older people's rights: Towards a UN convention a resource for promoting dialogue on creating a new UN convention on the rights of older persons. Available from: https://social.un.org/ageing-working-group/documents/Coalition%20to%20Strengthen%20the%20Rights%20of%20Older%20People.pdf

Hollomotz, A., 2009. Beyond 'vulnerability': An ecological model approach to conceptualizing risk of sexual violence against people with learning difficulties. *British Journal of Social Work*, *39*(1), pp. 99–112.

Joyce, K., Loe, M. and Diamond-Brown, L., 2015. Science, technology and ageing. In J. Twigg and W. Martin (eds.), *Routledge handbook of cultural gerontology*, p. 157. London, Routledge.

Knowles, M., 1973. *The adult learner: A neglected species*. Houston, TX, Gulf Publishing Company.

Lamb, S., 2015. Beyond the view of the west: Ageing and anthropology. In J. Twigg and W. Martin (eds.), *Cultural handbook of gerontology*, pp. 37–44. Abingdon, Oxon, Routledge.

Latham, J.R. and Barrett, C., 2015a. Appropriate bodies and other damn lies: Intersex ageing and aged care. *Australasian Journal on Ageing*, *34*(S2), pp. 19–20.

Latham, J.R. and Barrett, C., 2015b. *Gender is just a part of whom I am: Stories from trans Australians: Exploring the needs of trans people for health and aged care services*. La Trobe University, Melbourne.

Lottes, I.L., 2013. Sexual rights: Meanings, controversies, and sexual health promotion. *Journal of Sex Research*, *50*(3–4), pp. 367–391.

Lottes, I.L. and Adkins, C.W., 2003. The construction and psychometric properties of an instrument measuring support for sexual rights. *Journal of Sex Research*, *40*(3), pp. 286–295.

Mann, R., Horsley, P., Barrett, C. and Tinney, J., 2014. *Norma's project: A research study into the sexual assault of older women in Australia* (ARCSHS Monograph Series No. 98). Australian Research Centre in Sex, Health and Society, La Trobe University, Melbourne.

Marshall, B.L., 2015. Anti-ageing and identities. In *Routledge handbook of cultural gerontology*. Abingdon, Oxon, Routledge, pp. 210–216.

Ory, M., Hoffman, M.K., Hawkins, M., Sanner, B. and Mockenhaupt, R., 2003. Challenging aging stereotypes: Strategies for creating a more active society. *American Journal of Preventive Medicine*, *25*(3), pp. 164–171.

Parker, R.G., 2007. Sexuality, health, and human rights. *American Journal of Public Health*, *97*(6), p. 972.

Peel, N.M. and Warburton, J., 2009. Using senior volunteers as peer educators: What is the evidence of effectiveness in falls prevention? *Australasian Journal on Ageing*, *28*(1), pp. 7–11.

Plummer, K., 2001. The square of intimate citizenship: Some preliminary proposals. *Citizenship Studies*, *5*(3), pp. 237–253.

Plummer, K., 2005. Intimate citizenship in an unjust world. In M. Romero and E. Margolis (eds.), *The Blackwell companion to social inequalities*, pp. 75–99. New York, Wiley-Blackwell.

Plummer, K., 2010. The social reality of sexual rights. In P. Aggleton and R. Parker (eds.), *Routledge handbook of sexuality, health and rights*. Abingdon, Oxon, Routledge, pp. 45–55.

Plummer, K., 2012. Critical sexualities studies. In G. Ritzer (ed.), *The Wiley-Blackwell companion to sociology*, pp. 243–269. West Sussex, Wiley-Blackwell.

Plummer, K., 2013. Epilogue: A manifesto for critical humanism in sociology. In D. Nehring (ed.), *Sociology: An introductory textbook and reader*, pp. 489–517. New York: Pearson.

Richardson, D., 2000. Constructing sexual citizenship: Theorizing sexual rights. *Critical Social Policy*, *20*(1), pp. 105–135.

Rose, M.A., 1992. Evaluation of a peer-education program on heart disease prevention with older adults. *Public Health Nursing*, *9*(4), pp. 242–247.

Sheill, K., 2006. Sexual rights are human rights: But how can we convince the United Nations? *IDS Bulletin*, *37*(5), pp. 40–45.

Simon, W. and Gagnon, J., 2011. *Sexual conduct: The social sources of human sexuality*. New Brunswick, Transaction Publishers.

Turner, G. and Shepherd, J., 1999. A method in search of a theory: Peer education and health promotion. *Health Education Research*, *14*(2), pp. 235–247.

United Nations, 1983. Vienna international plan of action on ageing. Available from: www.un.org/es/globalissues/ageing/docs/vipaa.pdf

United Nations, 2002. Madrid international plan on action in ageing. Available from: www.un.org/esa/socdev/documents/ageing/MIPAA/political-declaration-en.pdf

United Nations, 2011. Follow-up to the second world assembly on ageing: Report of the secretary general. Available from: https://documents-dds-ny.un.org/doc/UNDOC/GEN/N11/428/83/PDF/N1142883.pdf?OpenElement

Wellings, K., Collumbien, M., Slaymaker, E., Singh, S., Hodges, Z., Patel, D. and Bajos, N., 2006. Sexual behaviour in context: A global perspective. *The Lancet*, *368*(9548), pp. 1706–1728.

World Association for Sexual Health, 1999. Declaration of sexual rights. Available from: www.worldsexology.org/wp-content/uploads/2013/08/declaration_of_sexual_rights_sep03_2014.pdf

World Health Organisation, 2002. Active ageing: A policy framework. Available from: http://apps.who.int/iris/bitstream/10665/67215/1/WHO_NMH_NPH_02.8.pdf

World Health Organisation, 2015. Data measuring the age-friendliness of cities: A guide to using core indicators. Available from: http://apps.who.int/iris/bitstream/10665/203830/1/9789241509695_eng.pdf

3

FRAMING THE SEXUAL RIGHTS OF OLDER HETEROSEXUAL WOMEN

Acknowledging diversity and change

Rachel Thorpe, Bianca Fileborn, and Laura Hurd Clarke

Introduction

Societal understandings of, and expectations about, sex in later life reflect and reinforce deeply entrenched ageist and sexist norms (Calasanti & Slevin 2001; Gott 2005; Higgs 1995). Sexuality is commonly conceptualised as a natural drive that is associated with reproduction, heterosexual intercourse and youthful bodies (Gott 2005). As such, cultural assumptions about what constitutes proper and legitimate sexuality exclude older women who have not traditionally been considered to be sexual citizens, irrespective of their sexual orientation (Gill 2007; Petchesky 2000; Richardson 2000). To date, the concerns of older women have been excluded from the sexual rights agenda (Plummer 2003; Petchesky 2000; Richardson 2000), and there is a dearth of research and theorizing about older women's sexuality. These omissions perhaps reflect the historical difficulty of conceptualising sexual rights in terms of positive sexuality rather than simply in terms of protection from rights abuses (Aboderin 2014; Petchesky 2000). However, such considerations are overdue, particularly given the realities of population ageing around the world. Indeed, the World Health Organization has predicted that by 2050, 16% of the global population will be over the age of 65, up from 8% in 2010 (World Health Organisation 2011). This pattern of global ageing is gendered, with women comprising 53% of adults aged 50 years and older and 59% of those aged 70 years and older (Stevens et al. 2013). Despite this gendered pattern of ageing, older women's sexuality is conspicuously absent from social policies and much of the extant research and theorizing. Reflecting this absence, institutionalised ageism and sexism operating within health care systems, social services, such as aged care, and culture more broadly continue to limit older women's ability to enjoy pleasurable and safe sexual experiences.

In this chapter, we consider which sexual rights are important for heterosexual older women from diverse backgrounds and how a sexual rights framework might be beneficial for the promotion and protection of the sexual expression of diverse older women. Using a feminist framework, we discuss the ways in which older women's sexual rights are shaped and constrained by structural factors such as age, ethnicity, gender norms, race, sexual orientation and social class. We examine the influence of gendered ageism and heterosexual norms on sexual rights as they apply in both the public and private domains, including sexual expression in the home, alone, with intimate partners and in institutional and aged care settings.

Conceptualising old age

Chronological age is important when considering sexuality, as with increasing age comes a greater likelihood that women will be living in institutional or aged care rather than in their own homes, as well as experiencing changes in opportunities for meeting partners and alterations in health, appearance and economic status. Each of these factors has potential implications for an older woman's sexual rights. For example, due to their longer life spans, as well as a variety of cultural factors, heterosexual women are more likely than men to be single in later life. As we discuss, this has implications for the social construction of older women as sexually desirable and desiring, as well as for their subjective sense of themselves as sexual (Connidis 2006; Hinchliff & Gott 2011).

We are also mindful of the role of generation in shaping the meanings of sexuality as we age (Plummer 2010; Rowntree 2014). Here, we refer to the influence of cultural changes over time in providing different opportunities for older women's (hetero)sexual practices, experiences of sexuality and of heterosexual relationships, and therefore for their sexual subjectivities. Such changes within Western countries include the separation of sex from marriage and reproduction, more liberal divorce laws and second-wave feminism (Hawkes 1996; Plummer 2010; Weeks 1985). These changes emerged roughly from the 1960s onwards, influencing, and being influenced by, various generations of women at different stages of their lives (Plummer 2010). For example, the notion of safe sex, emerging from the HIV/AIDS epidemic, is one that women born in the 1940s or earlier would not have been introduced to until mid-life or beyond. For a lot of women in long-term monogamous relationships, this concept was seen as irrelevant to their sexual practices and is something they and their male counterparts have only had to think about when negotiating new intimate relationships (Plummer 2010). As Chapter 9 raises, some do not consider the importance of safe sex for older adults even in the context of new relationships. These cultural changes are particularly significant for the sexualities of those who entered into sexual maturity during the 1960s and '70s – those who negotiated their early sexual relationships in this context and are currently negotiating sexuality in the context of ageing (Arber et al. 2007; Gott 2005; Loe 2004; Minichiello et al. 2005). Research findings suggest that those who came of age prior to these changes tend to discuss sex primarily within the context of monogamous, heterosexual marriage (Gott & Hinchliff 2003b, 2003c). Thus, there are likely to be starkly different experiences and attitudes towards sex within and between the different cohorts of women who currently make up the older population. More recent research reveals that older women are increasingly choosing not to marry, preferring to live alone, or to seek flexible relationships and living arrangements (Connidis 2006; Kirkman et al. 2015; Malta & Farquharson 2014; Rowntree 2014).

Similarly, the meanings attributed to old age must also be viewed as historically and culturally specific social constructions, particularly as a range of factors in addition to chronological age define later life (Gott 2005; Katz & Marshall 2003). For example, 'successful aging' (Rowe & Kahn 1997) increasingly equates optimal old age, often referred to as the 'third age' (Gilleard & Higgs 2007, p. 13), with health, activity and sexuality made possible through consumption. For women, this consumption centres primarily on their physical appearance, as they are expected to engage in beauty practices and interventions designed to make them look more youthful and sexually appealing (Calasanti & Slevin 2001; Hurd Clarke 2011; Slevin 2010). The positioning of sexuality as essential for positive ageing and citizenship claims simultaneously narrows the framing of sex as heterosexual intercourse (Katz & Marshall 2003) while also offering another lens through which to consider old age and sexual rights (Higgs 1995; Hockey & James 2003; Plummer 2003). Furthermore, the choices that are available to older people are greatly determined by income, health status and cultural context, despite often being considered as a matter of personal choice (Arber 2004; Twigg 2007). This neo-liberal individualisation of ageing has significant implications for the women who do not age successfully according to cultural standards and expectations. These women may engage in self-blame or be socially ostracised even as the role of structural and corporeal factors that shape our experiences of ageing and the ageing body are obscured or ignored. Notwithstanding the problems associated with these concepts, research has demonstrated that ideas regarding choosing how one ages, and having the freedom to express sexuality in older age, hold appeal for the current generation of older women (Rowntree 2014; Rowntree & Zufferey 2015).

The quantified (hetero)sexual self and sexual function in later life

Sex and sexuality tend to be framed in narrow, heteronormative ways within the bulk of current research on sex in later life. Existing quantitative research commonly measures the frequency of sexual activity with another person, with sexual activity usually referring to penetrative heterosexual intercourse (Gott 2005; Lindau & Gavrilova 2010). While the findings of such research have usefully countered assumptions of an asexual old age, they have also tended to narrowly define sexual activity as partnered sex, and use sexual frequency and physiological functioning as a proxy for sexual success in later life. The sexual experiences and subjectivities of single women are excluded under such an approach to sexuality, as are those of women who choose not to engage in sexual activity. Such quantitative research tells us little about how older women understand and experience their sexuality and sexual embodiment. For instance, to what extent are these experiences pleasurable or desirable for women? In what ways or to what extent does being sexual figure into an older woman's sense of identity? How do women negotiate sexual consent and sexual pleasure in partnered sexual activity?

The use of sexual function and frequency as a starting point for defining sexuality is underscored by ageism whereby youthful sexuality is used as the idealised standard (Gott 2005). We see this, for example, in the stereotype of the 'sexy senior' (the seemingly diametrically opposed counterpart to the 'asexual' senior [Gott 2005, p. 7], though both in fact reinforce the same problematic norms of youthful sexuality as the point of comparison for sexual success), who is able to overcome or avoid such physiological and biological changes as erectile dysfunction or vaginal dryness that often accompany ageing and thereby perform a youthful, healthy sexuality (Hinchliff & Gott 2008; Marshall & Katz 2012; Sandberg 2013). When considered through the lens of normative sexual function, the sexuality of older people, particularly when they do not fit the sexy senior ideal, tends to become classified as less than that of younger people (Bouman & Kleinplatz 2015). Associated with sexual decline, older bodies are positioned as being less capable than young bodies of 'normal' sexual functioning. Moreover, older women are frequently reported as having less interest in sex as compared to their male counterparts, particularly when they do not have a partner (Gott 2005; Lindau & Gavrilova 2010), and as having less sexual appeal as they increasingly deviate from normative youthful femininity (Vares 2009) – a position that is reinforced by cultural representations of ageing. These narratives have important implications for women's sense of themselves as sexual and the ways in which they express or enact their sexuality in later life. We return to this point in the proceeding section.

Sex and health

Due to the assumptions that sex and sexuality are 'naturally' less important for women as they age, older women are assumed to not need to receive information about sexuality or sexually transmitted infections (STIs), as such issues are considered irrelevant, if not inappropriate (Hinchliff 2015; Hirayama & Walker 2011; Hughes 2013; Ports et al. 2014). Ageing is generally associated with an increased prevalence of health problems, including chronic diseases and disabilities (Hurd Clarke & Bennett 2013; Hinchliff & Gott 2011; Villeneuve et al. 2015). Health status has been shown to influence the importance of sex to older people and the kinds of sex that they desire, with those reporting poor health being less likely to report an interest in sex (Gott & Hinchliff 2003b; Herbenick et al. 2010; Lindau & Gavrilova 2010). Having better health and greater interest in sex were also associated with having a partner, so that in such research older women were generally reported to be less sexually active than men simply by virtue of their age and gender (Herbenick et al. 2010; Lindau & Gavrilova 2010). However, research findings illustrate that even women with poorer health reported engaging in solo or partnered sexual activities, supporting the suggestion that even when sex may be a low priority, it is not necessarily unimportant to older women (Gott & Hinchliff 2003b; Herbenick et al. 2010).

Yet health care professionals, including primary care doctors, nurses and psychologists, are often reticent to talk to their older clients about sex and sexuality, while older women lament the lack of available resources on ageing and sexuality (Fileborn et al. 2015a; Flaget-Greener et al. 2015; Gott et al. 2004b; Hurd Clarke et al. 2014). A gap has been identified between the needs of older adults for information about sexuality and sexual health and the provision of such resources. The attitudes and beliefs of health care practitioners regarding the lack of importance of sex to older adults can prevent them from raising this topic with patients (Flaget-Greener et al. 2015; Gott & Hinchliff 2003a; Gott et al. 2004a; Gott et al. 2004b; Hinchliff & Gott 2011). These beliefs can also prevent older people from raising sex-related topics with health care practitioners (Gott & Hinchliff 2003a). In this way, older women's sexual rights – specifically the right to access "scientifically accurate and understandable information in relation to sexuality" – are jeopardised (World Association for Sexual Health [WAS] 1999). Research reveals that interventions designed to change the attitudes of practitioners towards older adults' sexuality, as well as sexuality education and training, could increase the likelihood of practitioners raising these topics with older patients, thereby improving the access of older people to up-to-date and unbiased information on sexual health (Flaget-Greener et al. 2015). Introducing the concept of sexual health knowledge and sexuality education as rights regardless of age, as stated in the WAS declaration (Chapter 2), during practitioner training could be a useful approach to take (WAS 1999).

Similar concerns have been raised in residential (institutional) aged care settings where some staff have been found to be dismissive or disapproving of the idea that older people might still be interested, let alone engaged, in sex and intimacy (Bauer et al. 2007; Hockey & James 1993). In two empirical studies, the majority of surveyed providers of residential aged care reported that they did not have a policy addressing sexuality or provide any written information for residents regarding intimacy and sexuality (Bauer et al. 2007; Doll 2013). Research findings show that staff members tend not to discuss the topic of sexuality with residents unless the resident raises it first, or staff perceive there to be a need for sexual expression, which typically only occurs in relation to married couples (Bauer et al. 2007; Rowntree & Zufferey 2015). This perspective privileges the sexuality of heterosexual married couples, rather than un-partnered or same-sex attracted women. Care facilities typically operate in a manner that provides residents with little privacy or control over when someone enters their room, affording little opportunity for sexual expression (Doll 2013; Heath 2011). For those residents in a partnered sexual relationship, the ability to share a bed or even a room is often not provided, again limiting the prospect of a sexual encounter and their right to privacy. We argue that it is imperative that residential care facilities respect and protect all older adults' rights to sexual expression (WAS 1999).

Certainly, consumers of institutional aged care have discussed the importance of privacy, autonomy and control, within a discourse of their right to choose to be sexually active (Rowntree & Zufferey 2015). These differences in understandings of sexuality between staff and residents highlight a need for policies and guidelines on sexuality and intimacy that take into account the perspectives, and rights, of older people (Bauer et al. 2007; Rowntree & Zufferey 2015). In addition to the right to privacy, the concept of sexual expression as a right could be incorporated into such policies and into staff training, as well as guidelines for determining the capacity of residents to consent to partnered sexual intimacy (Doll 2013). This would best be achieved through having older people involved in the development of guidelines and policies on sexuality, an approach that supports the WAS declaration's right to participate in public and political life. Aged care facilities also need to discuss their policies on sexuality and intimacy with residents upon their admission. Finally, beyond education and policy development, residential care facilities need to address spatial limitations and guarantee that privacy is offered to residents in appropriate and comfortable places as well as through the provision of meaningful and respectful opportunities.

Affirming older women's sexual rights

How can we rethink sexuality in later life in a way that does not negate older women's sexual rights and that avoids constructing the sexual functioning of older bodies as lesser or wanting in some respect? To what extent does such a construction reflect the embodied experiences of older women? Sandberg's (2013) concept of affirmative ageing provides a useful starting point. Instead of framing elder sexuality in relation to youthful sexuality, Sandberg argues that we should instead view the ageing process as the 'continuous production of difference' (p. 19). Such an approach flattens the sexual hierarchy, with youthful sexuality at its pinnacle, and demands that we view older people's sexuality on its own terms rather than in comparison to a youthful sexual norm. Importantly, Sandberg advocates for the recognition and acknowledgement of the specificities of the ageing body. According to this approach, it is not productive to deny or ignore changes in bodily functions or sensations, but neither is it helpful to view such bodily shifts as a decline or as automatically resulting in a less valuable sexual experience. Rather, Sandberg's concept opens up the possibility for considering different sexual experiences, which are shaped by gendered (and other structural) norms. While the sexual expression(s) and desire(s) of older women should not be identified as other to the norm, they also should not be uncritically accepted as some authentic expression of a true or essential sexual self.

Instead of neatly fitting the binary categories of the asexual older adult or the sexy senior, research investigating the meanings of sexuality and of sexual pleasure for older women illustrates that women's experiences of sex and sexual desire in later life are varied and complex (Fileborn et al. 2015a, 2015b; Gott 2005; Hurd Clarke 2006; Vares 2009). Older women have variably reported experiencing no sexual desire yet continuing to engage in partnered sex, experiencing desire and not having partnered or un-partnered sex, experiencing decreased desire as they age or, conversely, experiencing increased sexual desire as they age (often with the onset of a new romantic relationship), and many other fluid permutations of sexual activity, subjectivity and desire (Fileborn et al. 2015b; Loe 2004). For some women, sex becomes more pleasurable in later life as they have a stronger understanding of their own bodies and desires, are less willing to compromise on sexual satisfaction, and feel more able to negotiate their needs with their partner or to masturbate (Fileborn et al. 2015a, 2015b; Loe 2004). For others, penetrative sexual activity remains an expectation of partnered life and one from which they derive little personal sexual satisfaction – though it may be viewed as an altruistic act or as necessary for maintaining intimacy within a relationship. The cessation of both partnered and solo sexual activity, and the absence of sexual desire, can be a welcome relief for some women, whereas others may encounter this with a sense of sadness or loss (Fileborn et al. 2015a, 2015b; Loe 2004). The point here is not to provide an exhaustive description of older women's experiences and desires, or to construct certain experiences or desires as being more or less than others, but rather to illustrate the considerable diversity and fluidity that exists in women's experiences and reasons for engaging in sexual activity or not.

At the same time, research has highlighted the extent to which subjective sexual meanings and desires are socially and culturally constructed through the intersecting influences of sexism and ageism (Parker et al. 2000). Within women's own sexual and relationship histories what constitutes sex may have been shaped by gendered, sexist and ageist norms, in addition to the heterosexual institutions of marriage and motherhood, and religious mandates that sex is for the purpose of procreation. This holds important implications for women's right to be free from all forms of violence and coercion, as older women's ability to recognise and label experiences of sex as coerced (e.g. within marriage) may be constrained by these discourses (Chapter 8 of this volume explores this issue in further detail). While some older women hold diverse and inclusive definitions of what counts as sexual activity, for others (or for their partners) penetrative heterosexual intercourse is privileged as 'real' sex, whereas masturbation is viewed as a lesser form of sexual expression, reinforcing hierarchical understandings of sex (Fileborn et al. 2015a). These understandings limit the potential for sexual pleasure, particularly in the face of physiological changes that may make penetrative intercourse difficult, if not impossible, and the scarcity of available heterosexual partners, while also constructing older women's sexuality in response to a more pressing male sexual need and response (Fileborn et al. 2015a). This is not to suggest that penetrative sex is problematic in and of itself, but rather that the construction of penetrative sex as 'real' sex is narrow and serves to reinforce youthful models of sexuality rather than affirming the difference of older people's sexuality. Stereotypes of older individuals (and particularly older women) as asexual can also limit and shape the ways in which sexual desire is expressed or acknowledged and may lead to a downplaying of sexual desire or the belief that sex in later life is inappropriate (DeLamater & Koepsel 2015; Gray & Garcia 2012; Syme 2014; Trudel et al. 2010).

Research has also illustrated the role of these stereotypes in shaping women's interpretations of their bodies. Many women express dissatisfaction with the appearance of their older bodies due to age-related changes, such as weight gain and wrinkles, often citing young bodies as the point of comparison (Hurd 2000; Hurd Clarke 2011; Montemurro & Gillen 2013; Thorpe et al. 2015; Vares 2009). Older women generally find it difficult to ignore ageist and sexist values equating beauty with youth, and to negotiate a sense of self as both old and desirable in a context where they are surrounded by these very powerful images and messages. This is particularly the case for single women who desire intimacy but do not believe that a new partner would find them attractive (Hurd Clarke & Griffin 2008; Thorpe et al. 2015). Such findings reflect the lack of representations of older women, or of women showing the signs of age, as 'active, desiring sexual subjects' (Gill 2007, p. 152) in contemporary media culture. Yet research also demonstrates that some women become less concerned with conforming to youthful standards as they age (Tunaley et al. 1999). Old age can bring acceptance of bodily appearance as women construct positive, or contradictory, bodily meanings through drawing upon their biographies and embodied experiences (Holstein 2015; Krekula 2007; Thorpe et al. 2015). Such meanings may include disliking their ageing appearance in the mirror while expressing pride in the dressed body, appreciation of their health and physical abilities or satisfaction with the sensual qualities and appearance of their bodies during intimate encounters (Thorpe et al. 2015; Twigg 2013). Importantly, these findings remind us that the subjective experience of embodied old age is much more complex than women simply disliking their appearance and desiring to look younger, and that the notion of a sexual body includes different bodily qualities including touch, appearance, desire, as well as biographical dimensions. This multifaceted approach to the body can inform older women's right to claim sexual citizenship based upon a broad notion of sexuality, one that does not simply privilege a youthful appearance. Moreover, this understanding underscores the importance of including an analysis of gender in a sexual rights framework.

Conclusions

In this chapter we have explored the importance of sexual rights for older women's experiences of sexuality and embodied old age. Acknowledging the diverse and often contradictory meanings that are attached to older women's sexuality and ageing bodies, we have argued that it is imperative for health care professionals and institutions that provide aged care to acknowledge and foster the sexuality and healthy sexual expression of women in later life, whatever that means to individuals. The WAS declaration of sexual rights reaffirms that, "sexual health cannot be defined, understood or made operational without a broad understanding of sexuality" (WAS 1999). Adopting an inclusive perspective on sexuality is central to ensuring that older heterosexual women are able to enjoy sexual rights equally and without discrimination. With this in mind, we call for a countering of the ageist and sexist tendency for old age to be framed in terms of decline and asexuality as well as the equating of sexual ideals with youthful norms and assumptions. There is a paramount need to promote older women's right to a high level of sexual health and wellbeing, "including the possibility of pleasurable, satisfying and safe sexual experiences" (WAS 1999), should these be desired, as well as to consider the question of what pleasure is and how it is understood and constructed by older women. Enabling older women to enjoy their full sexual rights requires us to deconstruct and open up new possibilities or ways of thinking about sexual pleasure for all individuals.

In order for a rights-based framework to be actualised, the historical, cultural, contextual and relational influences on older women's lives must be taken into account. As such, the generationally specific understandings of sexuality should be tracked over time as new cohorts of women enter later life and both internalise and resist the cultural messages about the nature and role of sexuality in later life. The way in which we think about sexual rights will continue to change, for instance due to the expectations that successful sexuality brings for ageing women's sexual practices. Women will likely continue to be restrained in their sexual desires and expressions in the face of structural barriers and dominant normative constructions that devalue older women's lived experiences and construct limited normative sexual ideals and representations. Considering the ways in which these structures and norms may be challenged, disrupted and dismantled may be useful for setting out the claims that older women may make for positive sexual expression beyond these norms, whether they take these up or not.

Although we have advocated for the usefulness of a sexual rights approach throughout this chapter, it is important to consider the limitations of our argument. Notably, the bulk of research that we have considered here using an applied rights-based framework has been concerned with the experiences of white, middle- to upper-class women from Western countries. Yet, sexuality is conceptualised differently across different cultural contexts (Dune et al. 2015). As Parker (2009) highlights, 'many of the key categories and classifications that have been used to describe sexual life [in Western contexts] . . . are in fact far from universal or given in all cultural settings' (p. 256). Members of different ethnic or cultural groups are often sexualised in different ways – for instance, women of colour have often been depicted as 'hypersexual' (Miller 2005; Parker 2009). This is not to suggest, as Tamale (2008) argues, that we must view sexual rights as being *either* universal in their application or inappropriate for different cultures. Rather, 'cultures are fluid and interactive rather than distinct from each other. They are in constant flux, adapting and reforming' (Tamale 2008, p. 48). Sexual rights may have different implications or need to be employed in different ways both within and across different (sexual) cultures. Indeed, even within Western cultures, a sexual rights-based approach will hold varying levels of appropriateness and applicability, and this is liable to change over time and across contexts. Older women are constituted by diverse cultural, ethnic, social and other groups, and we cannot assume that a sexual rights framework can or should be applied in a uniform way. It is also important to acknowledge that the concept of rights is itself bound up in a particular political ideology – namely, male Western liberalism (Tamale 2008). Sexual rights are thus located within a particular political view of the world and bear particular cultural assumptions and norms. As such, careful consideration of whose interests this paradigm reflects and which ways of knowing and being in the world it propagates – and the extent to which these reflect the knowledge, values and experiences of older women – are needed.

This chapter has underscored the importance of acknowledging the diversity of sexuality and difference in the meanings of sexuality for older heterosexual women, as well as the kinds of sexual expression that women have a right to engage with and in which circumstances. We call for a sexual rights framework that is guided by women's own experiences and understandings about the significance of sexuality to them as they move through the life course, including the ways sexuality is negotiated by women of diverse cultures, classes and ages.

References

Aboderin, I 2014, 'Sexual and reproductive health and rights of older men and women: Addressing a policy blind spot', *Reproductive Health Matters*, vol. 22, no. 44, pp. 185–190.

Arber, S 2004, 'Gender, marital status, and ageing: Linking material, health, and social resources', *Journal of Aging Studies*, vol. 18, no. 1, pp. 91–108.

Arber, S, Andersson, L, & Hoff, A 2007, 'Changing approaches to gender and ageing', *Current Sociology*, vol. 55, no. 2, pp. 147–153.

Bauer, M, McAuliffe, L, & Nay, R 2007, 'Sexuality, health care and the older person: An overview of the literature', *International Journal of Older People Nursing*, vol. 2, no. 1, pp. 63–68.

Bouman, WP, & Kleinplatz, PJ 2015, 'Moving towards understanding greater diversity and fluidity of sexual expression of older people', *Sexual and Relationship Therapy*, vol. 30, no. 1, pp. 1–3.

Calasanti, T, & Slevin, K 2001, 'Sex, sexuality and old age', In: T Calasanti & K Slevin (eds.), *Gender, social inequalities and aging*. AltaMira Press, Walnut Creek, CA.

Connidis, IA 2006, 'Intimate relationships: Learning from later life experience', In: T Calasanti & K Slevin (eds.), *Age matters: Realigning feminist thinking*. Routledge, Milton Park, NY.

DeLamater, J, & Koepsel, E 2015, 'Relationships and sexual expression in later life: A biopsychosocial perspective', *Sexual and Relationship Therapy*, vol. 30, no. 1, pp. 37–59.

Doll, GM 2013, 'Sexuality in nursing homes. Practice and policy', *Journal of Gerontological Nursing*, vol. 39, no. 7, pp. 30–37.

Dune, T, Mapedzahama, V, Minichiello, V, Pitts, M, & Hawkes, G 2015, 'African migrant women's understanding and construction of sexuality in Australia', *Advances in Social Sciences Research Journal*, vol. 2, no. 2, pp. 38–50.

Fileborn, B, Thorpe, R, Hawkes, G, Minichiello, V, & Pitts, M 2015a, 'Sex and the (older) single girl: Experiences of sex and dating in later life', *Journal of Aging Studies*, vol. 33, pp. 67–75.

Fileborn, B, Thorpe, R, Hawkes, G, Minichiello, V, Pitts, M, & Dune, T 2015b, 'Sex, desire and pleasure: Considering the experiences of older Australian women', *Sexual and Relationship Therapy*, vol. 30, no. 1, pp. 117–130.

Flaget-Greener, M, Gonzalez, CA, & Sprankle, E 2015, 'Are sociodemographic characteristics, education and training, and attitudes toward older adults' sexuality predictive of willingness to assess sexual health in a sample of US psychologists?', *Sexual and Relationship Therapy*, vol. 30, no. 1, pp. 10–24.

Gill, R 2007, 'Postfeminist media culture: Elements of a sensibility', *European Journal of Cultural Studies*, vol. 10, no. 2, pp. 147–166.

Gilleard, C, & Higgs, P 2007, 'The third age and the baby boomers: Two approaches to the social structuring of later life', *International Journal of Ageing and Later Life*, vol. 2, no. 2, pp. 13–30.

Gott, M 2005, *Sexuality, sexual health and ageing*, Open University Press, Maidenhead, Berkshire.

Gott, M, Galena, E, Hinchliff, S, & Elford, H 2004a, 'Opening a can of worms': GP and practice nurse barriers to talking about sexual health in primary care', *Family Practice*, vol. 21, no. 11, pp. 528–536.

Gott, M, & Hinchliff, S 2003a, 'Barriers to seeking treatment for sexual problems in primary care: A qualitative study with older people', *Family Practice*, vol. 20, no. 6, pp. 690–695.

Gott, M, & Hinchliff, S 2003b, 'How important is sex in later life? The views of older people', *Social Science & Medicine*, vol. 56, no. 8, pp. 1617–1628.

Gott, M, & Hinchliff, S 2003c, 'Sex and ageing: A gendered issue', In: S Arber, K Davidson, & J Ginn (eds.), *Gender and ageing: Changing roles and relationships*. Open University Press, Maidenhead, Berkshire.

Gott, M, Hinchliff, S, & Galena, E 2004b, 'General practitioner attitudes to discussing sexual health issues with older people', *Social Science & Medicine*, vol. 58, no. 11, pp. 2093–2103.

Gray, P, & Garcia, J 2012, 'Ageing and human sexual behaviour: Biocultural perspectives _ a mini-review', *Gerontology*, vol. 58, no. 5, pp. 446–452.

Hawkes, G 1996, *A sociology of sex and sexuality*, Open University Press, Buckingham.

Heath, H 2011, 'Older people in care homes: Sexuality and intimate relationships', *Nursing Older People*, vol. 23, no. 6, pp. 14–20.

Herbenick, D, Reece, M, Schick, V, Sanders, SA, Dodge, B, & Fortenberry, JD 2010, 'Sexual behaviors, relationships, and perceived health status among adult women in the United States: Results from a national probability sample', *The Journal of Sexual Medicine*, vol. 7, pp. 277–290.

Higgs, P 1995, 'Citizenship and old age: The end of the road', *Ageing and Society*, vol. 15, no. 4, pp. 535–550.

Hinchliff, S 2015, 'When it comes to older people and sex, doctors put their heads in the sand', *The Conversation* [Online], viewed 20 June 2015, https://theconversation.com/when-it-comes-to-older-people-and-sex-doctors-put-their-heads-in-the-sand-43556

Hinchliff, S, & Gott, M 2008, 'Challenging social myths and stereotypes of women and aging: Heterosexual women talk about sex', *Journal of Women and Aging*, vol. 20, no. 2, pp. 65–81.

Hinchliff, S, & Gott, M 2011, 'Seeking medical help for sexual concerns in mid- and later life: A review of the literature', *The Journal of Sex Research*, vol. 48, no. 2–3, pp. 106–117.

Hirayama, R, & Walker, A 2011, 'Who helps older adults with sexual problems? Confidants versus physicians', *Journals of Gerontology: Psychological Sciences and Social Sciences*, vol. 66B, no. 1, pp. 109–118.

Hockey, J, & James, A 1993, *Growing up and growing old: Ageing and dependency in the life course*, Sage, London.

Hockey, J, & James, A 2003, *Social identities across the life course*, Palgrave Macmillan, Houndmills, Hampshire.

Holstein, M 2015, *Women in late life: Critical perspectives on gender and health*, Rowman & Littlefield, New York.

Hughes, A 2013, 'Mid-to-late-life women and sexual health: Communication with health care providers', *Family Medicine*, vol. 45, no. 4, pp. 252–256.

Hurd, LC 2000, 'Older women's body image and embodied experience: An exploration', *Journal of Women & Aging*, vol. 12, no. 3–4, pp. 77–97.

Hurd Clarke, L 2006, 'Older women and sexuality: Experiences in marital relationships across the life course', *Canadian Journal on Aging-Revue Canadienne Du Vieillissement*, vol. 25, no. 2, pp. 129–140.

Hurd Clarke, L 2011, *Facing age: Women growing older in anti-aging culture*, Rowman & Littlefield, Lanham, MD.

Hurd Clarke, L, & Bennett, EV 2013, '"You learn to live with all the things that are wrong with you": Gender and the experience of multiple chronic conditions in later life', *Ageing and Society*, vol. 33, no. 2, pp. 342–360.

Hurd Clarke, L, Bennett, EV, & Korotchenko, A 2014, 'Negotiating vulnerabilities: How older adults with multiple chronic conditions interact with physicians', *Canadian Journal on Aging*, vol. 33, no. 1, pp. 26–37.

Hurd Clarke, L, & Griffin, M 2008, 'Visible and invisible ageing: Beauty work as a response to ageism', *Ageing & Society*, vol. 28, no. 5, pp. 653–674.

Katz, S, & Marshall, B 2003, 'New sex for old: Lifestyle, consumerism, and the ethics of aging well', *Journal of Aging Studies*, vol. 17, no. 1, pp. 3–16.

Kirkman, L, Dickson-Smith, V, & Fox, C 2015, 'Midlife relationship diversity, sexual fluidity, wellbeing and sexual health from a rural perspective', *Rural Society*, vol. 24, no. 3, pp. 266–281.

Krekula, C 2007, 'The intersection of age and gender: Reworking gender theory and social gerontology', *Current Sociology*, vol. 55, no. 2, pp. 155–171.

Lindau, ST, & Gavrilova, N 2010, 'Sex, health, and years of sexually active life gained due to good health: Evidence from two US population based cross sectional surveys of ageing', *British Medical Journal*, vol. 340, viewed 15 December 2015, http://dx.doi.org/10.1136/bmj.c810

Loe, M 2004, 'Sex and the senior woman: Pleasure and danger in the viagra era', *Sexualities*, vol. 7, no. 3, pp. 303–326.

Malta, S, & Farquharson, K 2014, 'The initiation and progression of late-life romantic relationships', *Journal of Sociology*, vol. 50, no. 3, pp. 237–251.

Marshall, BL, & Katz, S 2012, 'The embodied life course: Post-ageism or the renaturalization of gender', *Societies*, vol. 2, no. 4, pp. 222–234.

Miller, A 2005, 'Sexual rights, conceptual advances: Tensions in debate', *Sexual, reproductive & human rights seminar, organised by C.L.A.D.E.M.*, Lima.

Minichiello, V, Ackling, S, Bourne, C, & Plummer, D 2005, 'Sexuality, sexual intimacy and sexual health in later life', In: V Minichiello & I Coulson (eds.), *Contemporary issues in gerontology: Promoting positive ageing*. Allen and Unwin, Crows Nest, NSW.

Montemurro, B, & Gillen, MM 2013, 'Wrinkles and sagging flesh: Exploring transformations in women's sexual body image', *Journal of Women and Aging*, vol. 25, no. 1, pp. 3–23.

Parker, R 2009, 'Sexuality, culture and society: Shifting paradigms in sexuality research', *Culture, Health & Sexuality*, vol. 11, no. 3, pp. 251–266.

Parker, R, Barbosa, RM, & Aggleton, P 2000, *Framing the sexual subject: The politics of gender, sexuality and power*, University of California Press, Berkeley.

Petchesky, RP 2000, 'Sexual rights: Inventing a concept, mapping an international practice', In: R Parker, RM Barbosa & P Aggleton (eds.), *Framing the sexual subject: The politics of gender, sexuality and power*. University of California Press, Berkeley.

Plummer, K 2003, *Intimate citizenship: Private decisions and public dialogues*, University of Washington Press, Seattle and London.

Plummer, K 2010, 'Generational sexualities, subterranean traditions, and the hauntings of the sexual world: Some preliminary remarks', *Symbolic Interaction*, vol. 33, no. 2, pp. 163–190.

Ports, KA, Barnack-Tavlaris, JL, Syme, ML, Perera, RA, & Lafata, JE 2014, 'Sexual health discussions with older adult patients during periodic health exams', *The Journal of Sexual Medicine*, vol. 11, no. 4, pp. 901–908.

Richardson, D 2000, *Rethinking sexuality*, Sage, London.

Rowe, JW, & Kahn, RL 1997, 'Successful aging', *The Gerontologist*, vol. 37, no. 4, pp. 433–440.

Rowntree, MR 2014, 'Comfortable in my own skin: A new form of sexual freedom for ageing baby boomers', *Journal of Aging Studies*, vol. 31, pp. 150–158.

Rowntree, MR, & Zufferey, C 2015, 'Need or right: Sexual expression and intimacy in aged care', *Journal of Aging Studies*, vol. 35, pp. 20–25.

Sandberg, L 2013, 'Affirmative old age: The ageing body and feminist theories on difference', *International Journal of Aging and Later Life*, vol. 8, no. 1, pp. 11–40.

Slevin, KF 2010, 'If I had lots of money . . . I'd have a body makeover: Managing the aging body', *Social Forces*, vol. 88, no. 3, pp. 1003–1020.

Stevens, GA, Mathers, CD, & Beard, JR 2013, *Global mortality trends and patterns in older women*, Bull World Health Organisation, vol. 91, pp. 630–631.

Syme, ML 2014, 'The evolving concept of older sexual behaviour and its benefits', *Generations*, vol. 38, no. 1, pp. 35–41.

Tamale, S 2008, 'The right to culture and the culture of rights: A critical perspective on women's sexual rights in Africa', *Feminist Legal Studies*, vol. 16, pp. 47–69.

Thorpe, R, Fileborn, B, Hawkes, G, Pitts, M, & Minichiello, V 2015, 'Old and desirable: Older women's accounts of ageing bodies in intimate relationships', *Sexual and Relationship Therapy*, vol. 30, no. 1, pp. 156–166.

Trudel, G, Turgeon, L, & Piché, L 2010, 'Marital and sexual aspects of old age', *Sexual and Relationship Therapy*, vol. 25, no. 3, pp. 316–341.

Tunaley, JR, Walsh, S, & Nicolson, P 1999, '"I'm not bad for my age": The meaning of body size and eating in the lives of older women', *Ageing & Society*, vol. 19, no. 6, pp. 741–759.

Twigg, J 2007, 'Clothing, age and the body: A critical review', *Ageing & Society*, vol. 27, no. 2, pp. 285–305.

Twigg, J 2013, *Fashion and age: Dress, the body and later life*, Bloomsbury, London.

Vares, T 2009, 'Reading the "sexy oldie": Gender, age(ing) and embodiment', *Sexualities*, vol. 12, no. 4, pp. 503–524.

Villeneuve, L, Trudel, G, Dargis, L, Preville, M, Boyer, R, & Begin, J 2015, 'The influence of health over time on psychological distress among older couples: The moderating role of marital functioning', *Sexual and Relationship Therapy*, vol. 30, no. 1, pp. 60–77.

Weeks, J 1985, *Sexuality and its discontents: Meanings, myths and modern sexualities*, Routledge and Kegan Paul plc, London.

World Health Organisation 2011, Global Health and Aging, NIH Publication no. 11-7737, viewed 18 July 2017, http://www.who.int/ageing/publications/global_health.pdf

4

OLDER MEN'S EXPERIENCES OF SEXUALITY AND THEIR RELEVANCE FOR SEXUAL RIGHTS

Hans Wiggo Kristiansen and Linn J. Sandberg

Introduction

The sexualities of older men are ambiguous and ridden with contradictions. Some men's sexual attractiveness is more readily recognised, also as they become older. This is, for example, seen in the case of the iconic actor Sean Connery, who seems to be a continuous lure to (younger) women, and when featuring in a Dewar's Whisky commercial at age 74 securely states: "some age, others mature" (Dewar's commercial 2004). In their everyday lives, however, men may experience anxieties about their desirability and abilities to perform sexually as they grow older. Notably, men's experiences of sexuality in later life are shaped by context and by differences such as sexual orientation and experiences of illness and disability. In terms of gender, older men's sexualities are often prioritized at the expense of older women (Calasanti, Slevin & King 2006; Loe 2004). This has not least become visible in the "Viagra era," where the introduction of pharmaceuticals aiming to restore or enhance men's sexual potency have further bolstered the significance of the erect penis for pleasurable sex, also in later life (Loe 2004; Marshall 2006, 2010; Marshall & Katz 2002; Potts et al. 2006; Tiefer 2006), as is discussed in Chapter 10. Still the impact of ageism shapes the experiences of later-life sexuality, for both men and women, positioning older people as undesirable and/or undesiring and thus continuously overlooked in discussions of sexuality and sexual rights.

Given the ambiguous and contradictory status of older men's sexualities, how then is the matter of sexual rights pertinent to the sexualities of older men? In this chapter we explore how men, heterosexual as well as gay and bisexual, experience their sexuality in later life to further consider how sexual rights can be understood in relation to men, masculinities, ageing and sexuality. Any discussion of sexual rights should take as its point of departure the actual experiences of older men, and comparing heterosexual and non-heterosexual men's challenges and concerns is a necessary precursor to articulating and discussing sexual rights. The gendered body is also an ageing body and a sexually oriented body, to paraphrase Marshall and Katz (2002), and looking more closely at the intersections of gender, age and sexual orientation may enable us to interrogate the simultaneous vulnerability and privilege that characterizes older men's sexualities. In some ways, dominant discourses on gender and sexuality privilege all men, regardless of sexual orientation. In other ways, the situation for older heterosexual men differs fundamentally from that of older gay and bisexual men.

Thus, in contrast to most research on ageing and sexuality, this chapter attempts to provide a common framework for understanding the experiences of heterosexual *and* non-heterosexual men. Comparing experiences of sexuality among heterosexual, gay and bisexual older men is a way to challenge heteronormative assumptions and highlight how the position of older gay and bisexual men with respect to sexual rights is still marginal compared to that of older heterosexual men. Still, it is worth asking if it is possible to identify common concerns and coping strategies among older men, regardless of their sexual orientation. Is the ageism that older heterosexual men experience when trying to live full sexual lives similar to that experienced by non-heterosexual men? It should be noted, however, that the chapter focuses on cis-identified men (i.e. men who identify with the biological sex they were assigned at birth), and that this reflects the sample of the majority of the studies on older men and sexuality to date. For a discussion of the experiences of trans- and intersex people, see Chapters 6 and 7 in this volume.

In this chapter we highlight older men's diverse experiences and attitudes toward sexuality in later life and how these can be understood and translated into improved understanding of their sexual rights. Sexuality is discussed as sexual practice in a wide sense, but also in terms of sexual desire and experiences of one's own sexual desirability. Three ways in which men relate to sexuality in later life are elaborated on in the following: (1) aspirations to continued sexual assertion, potency and performance; (2) renouncing sexuality; and (3) redefining and broadening concepts of sex and sexuality. These three approaches reflect a diversity of experiences of sexuality that go beyond simplistic definitions of ageing male sexuality. It is important to note that these approaches are not typologies specific to certain men, but that the same men could, for example, simultaneously attempt to regain potency and engage in a redefinition of sexual practice beyond phallic sexuality. Furthermore, these approaches may be encountered among both men who identify as heterosexuals and men who identify as gay or bisexual, although they may resonate differently depending on sexual orientation. Our discussion is based on existing international literature on the sexualities of ageing men. More specific examples are drawn from two empirical studies on the narratives of intimacy and sexuality among old Swedish heterosexual men (Sandberg 2011) and one on the life stories of ageing gay men in Norway (Kristiansen 2004a, 2008).

Aspirations to continued sexual assertion, potency and performance

Even though older men in existing studies on sexuality tend to indicate that they are less sexually active than they were in their younger years, and that sexual desire may diminish as one ages, there are also examples of how men continue to assert themselves sexually. For some, this may mean stressing a continued desire for sex or feeling attracted to women (Sandberg 2011). For gay men in particular, sexual assertion may also involve seeking new sexual partners and casual sexual encounters, often in cross-generational sexual relationships (Kristiansen 2004a; Suen 2015). For example, in Kristiansen's (2004a) ethnographic study with 23 Norwegian gay men aged 60 to 82, Trygve (a participant in his early seventies) described how he is continuously sexually active and desirable as an older man:

> There are a whole lot of young men who like grown-up men. I have never in my life had more opportunity than after I rounded 60 and up till now. I still get off with them, no problem. And I used to think that it was weird, but I've learned that there are actually a whole lot who like grown-up, older men.

Other researchers note that there are many venues within gay subcultures, such as leather and bear clubs, where the middle-aged and older male bodies and the experience of older gay men is honoured and even fetishized (Wierzalis et al. 2006; Slevin & Linneman 2010; Hennen 2008). Some talk about the existence of a distinct "Daddy" culture within the wider gay subculture, and also the resurgence and emergence of the older man in gay pornography (Mercer 2014).

As the Western sexual script on male sexuality is highly focused on erectile function, men's continued sexual assertion is often tied to maintaining potency. This was reflected in Sandberg's (2011) study on older heterosexual men, where 22 Swedish men aged 67 to 87 participated through interviews and/or 'body diaries'. Axel, an 83-year-old interviewee, highlighted the need for potency as a central part of sexual satisfaction by describing penile-vaginal penetrative sex as the "frosting on the cake". Axel also reflected the common discourse that men need potency to be men at all:

> If I'd stop being with her that I'm seeing now, whom I've been seeing for eleven years, and she'd tell [people] that I couldn't get a hard-on, that would be absolutely terrible for me. A man should have potency. Of course those who are younger are generally saying old geezers and old crones shouldn't do those kinds of things.

In this extract, Axel alludes to a discourse of asexual old age but contravenes it by pointing to the significance of potency for him, also as an older man. In the cases where men are highly invested in the idea of potency as necessary to male identity, changes in erectile function, which are commonplace to men as they age, could be experienced as a significant hardship and a "blow to masculinity" (Sandberg 2011; Gledhill & Schweitzer 2014). In a qualitative study by Gledhill and Schweitzer (2014) involving six heterosexual men aged 65 to 84, erectile dysfunctions were associated with stress and described as a devastating and frustrating experience. The men in this study experienced erectile dysfunction as troubling because of concerns with not being able to satisfy their partners. Similar results are expanded on by Sandberg (2011). Several of Sandberg's interviewees expressed fears that a female partner may become disappointed and dissatisfied if he was unable to get an erection and perform subsequent penetration. This was most troublesome for men who were not in relationships and where meeting new partners could involve a 'failed' performance.

A strong imperative within the narratives of Sandberg's study was that men were "responsible" for women's sexual satisfaction, a form of "sexual breadwinner model" where heterosexual men were expected to provide for their female partners. Although few men in Sandberg's study provided vague and unconfirmed anecdotes of women being disappointed or dissatisfied with men's inabilities to perform an erection, a coital imperative and a strong reliance on a "phallogocentric model of sex" pervaded the men's narratives (Sandberg 2011; Oliffe 2005). The idea of men as responsible for women's sexual pleasure, most notably through the delivery of firm erections, also reflects the idea of sexual activity as duty in relationships. In the quantitative US study *Sex, Romance, and Relationships: 2009 AARP Survey of Midlife and Older Adults*, surveying 1,670 adults older than age 45, 61% of males older than 70 agreed that "sexual activity is a duty to one's spouse/partner" (Fisher 2010, p. 20). This attitude in combination with a strong coital imperative is thus shaping some heterosexual men's experiences of later-life sexuality.

The pervasive understanding of later life as a time of asexuality has increasingly been challenged by understandings of sexuality as life-long and part of healthy ageing (Sandberg 2016). This is linked to the assumption that to remain sexually active is to remain young. Or, to quote an American self-help manual: "In short, you don't stop having sex because you get old, you get old because you stop having sex" (Danoff 1993, pp. 155–156, quoted in Marshall & Katz 2002, p. 62). As discussed by Calasanti and King (2005), media imagery is increasingly presenting old men as "playing hard" and "staying hard", where continued physical performance and activity is combined with sustained sexual performance and ability. Discourses of successful ageing are thus increasingly focused on sex for life, but simultaneously equate continued sexuality narrowly with men's abilities to retain erections. The advent of Viagra and other potency-enhancing drugs has been significant to this shift in discourse. However, if older men's experiences of sexuality are directed by discourses of being a man through sexual assertiveness and the ability to have an erection, then Viagra and other drugs for erectile function may put further pressure on men to perform sexually as they age and for heterosexual men to "provide" sexual satisfaction for women, in line with narrow standards of masculine sexuality. Notably, the anxieties associated with erectile changes seem to differ between heterosexual and non-heterosexual men. According to Lyons et al. (2015), the feeling of being less desirable now that they were older, and decreased confidence in their own appearance, seemed to be more important to older gay men than concerns about their own loss of sexual desire or potency.

Continued sexual activity may be an important aspect of positive ageing for heterosexual and non-heterosexual men alike, although the significance of erectile function may vary. In terms of sexual rights, 'the right to the highest attainable standard of health including sexual health' is of clear relevance to older men as men's bodily ageing, and in particular changes in erectile function, may impact on health and well-being. As highlighted in Chapter 10, the provision of pharmaceuticals for potency could thus be understood as optimizing the right to sexual health as erectile dysfunction may cause distress for some men, and also links to the 'right to enjoy the benefits of scientific progress'. From this perspective, advancements in medicine may benefit older men by helping them to regain their erections. However, medical solutions may also function as unfulfilled promises for some men for whom these treatments do not work, causing even further stress and anxiety, not least in cases where heterosexual men are invested in ideas of providing sexually for their partners. As such, they may serve to reinforce a phallic imperative and normative masculinity, which causes harm to men and their partners. From this perspective, the right to information and sexual education to challenge normative masculinity may be just as central in terms of sexual rights.

A sexual rights perspective on older men's sexualities should also consider how men, who wish to continue to assert themselves sexually as they age, negotiate negative and degrading stereotypes such as that of 'dirty old men', which may impact negatively on self-esteem and mental health. Next we will discuss how men's renunciations of sexuality may both be a reflection of ageist stereotypes of dirty old men and reflections of a positive experience of less strong sexual desires as one ages.

Renouncing sexuality: loss of desire or loss of desirability

If ageing and old age are experienced as threats to masculinity and the assertion of sexuality is perceived as a way of buttressing a masculine self, then a fading of sexual desire may be difficult to accept and even harder to articulate. If "sex for life" is increasingly becoming part of healthy and successful ageing, it may be increasingly difficult to discuss experiences of decline in desire as a natural part of ageing experiences, for both men and women.

There are, however, examples of renunciations of sexuality among both heterosexual and non-heterosexual men. These renunciations are interesting because they point to how men may handle and negotiate gender and age norms in different ways. There are also differences between men with respect to whether the renunciations of sexuality are voluntary and experienced as a freedom or if they were felt as involuntary. Understanding these differences may assist us in understanding the sexual rights of older men.

Both heterosexual and non-heterosexual men report that sexual interest and desire may decline as one ages. This may reflect both the understanding of biological ageing and cultural norms and expectations where ageing with dignity involved being less sexually active and desirable (Sandberg 2011; Wentzell 2011; Kristiansen 2004a, 2004b, 2013; Lyons et al. 2015). Several studies point to gay communities as obsessed with youth and youthful standards of beauty and that older gay and bisexual men may feel marginalized within the "bar scene", which for many is a predominant context for sexual contacts (Slevin & Linneman 2010; Lyons et al. 2015). Older gay and bisexual men may have internalized ageist perceptions of their sexuality and thus feel less desirable. The reasons that many men in Kristiansen's study gave for not continuing to visit venues such as bars, bath houses and other cruising areas (i.e. public areas where people go to look for a sexual partner) was not that they would be unable to *act* (have sex) in appropriate ways with a potential partner. Instead, it was the fear that they would *look* stupid, which was linked to the negative stereotype of the 'pathetic and unappetizing older homosexual' on the prowl for young men. This stereotype persists alongside the more affirming images of older gay and bisexual men discussed earlier. Kristiansen's interview with Sigurd, a man aged over 80, narrates a very active sexual life in midlife, after having divorced his wife, where he had multiple partners. However, at the time of the interview he considered his sex life to be over:

> But now I've given it all up. And I prayed to Our Lord for that, because I've always felt disgusted by those old homosexuals who hang out by the urinals and . . . like this (opens his mouth and stares out into the air with widely opened eyes). Yes. And I didn't want to become like that. So I've prayed for that every night. I started doing that when I passed 70, or at least at 75. And he has answered my prayers: I feel no [desire]. I have given it up [. . .] Oh no, I've never been a nice boy. I've had my share. But as I tell my friends: I will age with dignity.

As Kristiansen (2013) argues, Sigurd's belief that his sexual life had ended seemed to be more about presenting himself as a respectable older man than fully reflecting his loss of desire for sex. Several other older gay men in this study expressed relief at being beyond sexual desire and said that they felt more relaxed and at ease now that their sexual desire was a thing of the past.

Compared to studies of non-heterosexual older men, few of the heterosexual men in Sandberg's (2011) study reiterate negative stereotypes of "dirty old men" and of the older man as undesirable. Still there are examples of how old-age nega-tivity and ageist stereotypes may shape older heterosexual men's experiences of sexuality. When asked about what one may find attractive in him, Ingvar laughed and pointed at a photo of himself standing by a sports car and said, "Look at this sports car, a lot of women are drawn to that". His joking response to the question suggests that his potential attractiveness lay in his material possession rather than in himself as a person. This, in combination with how he recurrently refers to himself as an "old geezer" and that not many women are drawn to old men like himself, seem to shape his experiences of sexual desire. Even though he reported that he still had an interest in women and that this was "natural to men", he simultaneously said that he was not "particularly attracted to sex". Ingvar's life situation, being recently widowed combined with previous experiences of erectile dysfunction, is likely to impact on his experiences of sexual desire.

For the few men in Sandberg's study who actually articulated a loss of sexual desire, this was mostly made sense of in relation to illnesses such as prostate cancer and medical treatments thereof. Even for these men, however, the loss of sexual desire was experienced as an "odd feeling" that risked disrupting their gendered identity (Sandberg 2013). Men tended to solve this problem by pointing to their strong sexual desires to women in the past, to reinstate an intelligibly heterosexual masculine life course. A lack or loss of desire may be experienced as less damaging to the subjectivity of gay and bisexual men, who most of their adult lives have been living with a stigmatized sexual identity that excludes them from the category of "real men" in the first place.

Although we have so far primarily discussed renunciation of sex as negative experiences, the loss of an earlier strong sexual desire could also be experienced as a freedom for older men. In Kristiansen's (2013) study, Willy, a gay man in his early seventies who in his younger days had made numerous sexual contacts in public restrooms and parks in Oslo, expressed that he was relieved that the urge for sex was gone, a fact he attributed to his diabetes:

> So I just want to live in peace. That's all that matters to me now. I don't have any desire. I might look at a pretty boy, just like I look at a flower. But I no longer run after him or try to make a pass at him.

This expression of relief at no longer having to chase casual sex may be more pertinent to gay and bisexual men who have led very active sexual lives and sought many casual sexual encounters. Similarly, heterosexual men describe how the significance of intimacy and touch increases as they age and how a more serene sexual desire opens up to more diverse experiences of pleasure (Potts et al. 2006; Sandberg 2011).

Whether different men's renunciations of sex are voluntary or not, and whether the reported loss of sexual desire is due to biological changes (e.g. declines in testosterone) or complying with cultural norms is difficult to know. Context, including sexual biographies of the life course, is likely to impact greatly on how men handle and approach sexuality and sexual desire as they age. Some gay and bisexual men, who experience late-onset "sexual blooming" after having lived for many years in heterosexual marriages, may feel less inclined to terminate their sexual lives in older years than those who have had a more continuous sexual life course. For heterosexual men, widowhood can impact on how sexual desire becomes possible. Some widowers may experience ongoing grief and feelings of guilt after meeting a new partner (Smith 2013). Long-term married men may also have lived as "married celibates" where sexual activities ceased many years ago or where they had little sexual experience before marriage, which may impact on their confidence (Smith 2013, p. 71). Renouncing sexuality could thus be an expression of this life situation.

In terms of sexual rights, older men's renunciation of sexuality must simultaneously be understood as a possible freedom from pressure to perform sexually and to maintain a masculine identity, and an internalization of depreciative stereotypes of older men as non-desirable and whose sexual desires are inappropriate. We believe that challenging the discourses of an asexual old age is an important aspect of advancing the sexual rights of older people. The construction of older men's sexuality as "dirty" or inappropriate may be a hindrance to the pursuit of a sexually pleasurable later life and lead some men to give up on sexuality. For some gay and bisexual men, the intersection of homophobia and ageism impact in particularly vicious ways through negative stereotyping. Advancing the sexual rights of "non-discrimination and equality" and "autonomy and bodily integrity" of older men thus must involve a dual confrontation of these structures. Still, considering how normative masculinity dictates that men are always sexually willing, some older men's embracing of asexuality may in fact be a strategy to depart from gendered expectations and not always signs of neither pathology nor internalized ageism.

The feeling of becoming invisible as a sexual object and sexual subject is often mentioned by older men, gay or bisexual as well as heterosexual, as seen in the previous discussion. The sexual rights discourse does not fully cover these experiences, and sexual rights could thus be supplemented with the concept of "sexual dignity", which refers to a person's sense of self-respect or self-worth in interaction with others. Lottes (2013 with reference to Horton 2004) outlines four main categories of dignity violations, all of which are relevant to sexual dignity. The first two violations "being ignored or insufficiently acknowledged" and "being seen, but only as member of a group", touch upon the right to equality and non-discrimination, and specifically on the experience of being excluded from the realm of the sexual for being considered "old".

Redefining and broadening concepts of sex

Discussions on sexuality and ageing, both in the scientific literature and public discourses, have mainly focused on sexuality in terms of dysfunctions and problems. In terms of older men, this has involved a significant focus on erectile dysfunction, which is sometimes posited as a "fate worse than death" (Tiefer 2004, p. 254). Although, as discussed earlier, problems with erectile function may be experienced as challenging for men in terms of masculinity, qualitative studies in particular have also suggested that the ageing of bodies and changing life circumstances in later life may incite redefinitions of sex and a broadening of what counts as pleasurable sex and intimacy.

For some heterosexual men, experiences of ageing embodiment, including but not limited to a decline in erectile function, meant an increasing focus on wider pleasures, including touch and non-coital sex (Hughes 2011; Potts et al. 2006; Sandberg 2011). Interviewees in Potts and colleagues' (2006, p. 316) study in New Zealand, involving 12 men aged 54 to 70, expressed that where sex earlier in life was more about "empty out and move on", "a 'selfish' penis-focused sex", sexuality in mid-life and beyond involved shifting focus to a wider array of non-penile pleasures. These results resonate with Sandberg's study (2011), where heterosexual men with increasing experience and changing bodies claimed to enjoy the "whole of the body" to a greater extent than when younger. Sexual satisfaction was thus not dependent on the functioning of the penis (Fisher 2010; Hughes 2011). Importantly, and as Sandberg (2011) argues, the same men who initially experienced impotence as a disaster may find coping strategies and develop new definitions of sex that are not necessarily experienced as substitutes for penetrative sex. In Ménard and colleagues' (2015) study, which involved 30 heterosexual men and women aged 60 to 82 years who identified as having "great sex" in later life, the researchers argue that unlearning and overcoming earlier narrow definitions of sex was central to optimal sex. One participant, an older man who lived with a neurodegenerative disease, expressed that his "previous definitions of sex weren't working", and he consequently started experimenting and eventually experienced that:

> Sex was much more intense than it ever was before. And I like that, even though, I mean, even though I still wasn't, um, um, having erections or orgasms myself, but the whole experience as a whole was, I thought, was much greater than anything I had back then.
>
> *(Ménard et al. 2015, p. 84)*

Similar intents on broadening the definition of sex could also be found among older gay and bisexual men who were living in relationships with their male partner. Åge, one of the older gay men in Kristiansen's study, who had lived with his 10-years-older partner Knut for more than 40 years, related how they had stopped having sex 10 years earlier. Åge did not express regret at the fact that the sexual part of their relationship was over. "When you're too old you're too old, and that's it", he said. But it was much harder for him to accept that his partner stopped touching him. He had gotten so used to his partner patting his back or bottom in passing, while asking him: "How are you today, my dear?" In connection with himself falling ill with cancer, Åge confronted his partner with this concern. During one of their visits to the hospital, the couple went on a ride in their car. Åge touched his partner Knut on his cheek and told him that they had to start touching each other again:

> And I think he was extremely grateful that I brought it up, because it was as if he had closed himself up, somehow, and was unable to unlock himself. But I could [unlock him]. And that was very rewarding.

Sandberg (2011) suggests that intimacy and touch destabilize boundaries between the sexual and the non- or even asexual and implode the very category of sexuality. In the previous example, resuming the everyday practice of touching each other's bodies was considered a renewal of the former sexual bond between the two men, confirming anew their couple relationship.

Moreover, for older gay and bisexual men, sex is often redefined away from hetero-masculine expectations at a much earlier stage in their life courses, namely when they started to engage in sexual relations with other men. In contrast, hetero-sexual men may experience de-masculinization for perhaps the first time in their lives as they age (Meadows & Davidson 2006). Thus, older gay and bisexual men may indeed be ahead of their heterosexual peers in some ways as they face the daily challenges of inhabiting older bodies. Engaging in male-to-male sexual practice (e.g. having and enjoying penetrative sex in the receptive role or satisfying a partner orally) is fully compatible with not being able to sustain an erection. Men who engage in impersonal sexual encounters in cruising areas, for instance, may change roles as they age, as described in Laud Humphreys' classic *Tearoom Trade* (1970). In such settings, there is often no expectation of reciprocity in sexual transactions, and an older man may enjoy "servicing" other men without the expectation of them returning the service (see also Cohler 2004).

Moreover, the non-phallic sexual practices that some older men, both hetero-sexual and non-heterosexual, are able to develop could be seen as inspirational for challenging normative masculine sexuality. Making available coping strategies and ways of handling changing sexual functions may be just as important in the pursuit of sexual health for older men as is the provision of medical cures. There may be opportunities for heterosexual men to learn from gay and bisexual men to take a more passive role and explore new erogenous zones of the body. Gay and bisexual men frequently report a greater sense of freedom from cultural norms. This may mean a highly adaptive flexibility in terms of which roles and role expectations are "acceptable" (Wahler & Gabbay 1997, p. 14). Moreover, for heterosexual older couples, the disruption of a coital imperative may also benefit and empower female partners sexually, giving them more agency and freedom to explore new aspects of their own sexuality (Fileborn et al. 2015; McCarthy, Farr & McDonald 2013; Potts et al. 2003).

Earlier we discussed how being able to be continually active through penetrative sex could be an important aspect of sexual health and well-being for older men and as such considered a sexual right. But the empirical studies discussed previously, which point to the significance of broadening and redefining sexual practices beyond erections and penetrative sex, also indicate that rights to information and sexual education may be just as important in order to help men enjoy sexual practices beyond (hetero)normative masculinity, with a partner or by oneself. The third sexual right (see Chapter 2) relates to autonomy and bodily integrity and states that "Older people have the right to control and decide freely on matters related to their sexuality and their body. This includes the choices of sexual behaviours, practices, partners and relationships with due regard to the rights of others". In this context, it could read as the possibility for older men to find pleasurable practices in the widest possible (consensual) sense, not being limited by coital imperatives or penile-focused sex.

Concluding remarks: towards an intersectional approach to older men's sexual rights

In this chapter we have discussed the sexual rights of older men, taking older men's own experiences as expressed in qualitative studies as our point of departure. Our discussion points to a diversity of attitudes and experiences of sexuality among older men, and there were both similarities and differences between heterosexual and non-heterosexual men. Men expressed the desire for continued sexual activity, but some had given up sexuality in later life. Concern was expressed about changes in erectile function and the need to broaden and negotiate sexual repertoires as they were ageing. To conclude, we will summarize the main social and cultural hindrances to older men pursuing a satisfying, safe and pleasurable sexual life, but also what the possibilities may be in terms of supporting older men's sexual rights.

As we note in the introduction, in terms of gender, men's sexualities are privileged in many respects. Still, masculinity may also be a hindrance for men to obtain optimal sexual pleasure and satisfaction, in particular for older men who are unable to live up to normative gendered expectations as they are ageing. Discourses of men as always sexually willing and the significance of the erection for the maintenance of masculinity may have detrimental effects on the sexual health and well-being of men as they age. Sexual rights of older men should thus take masculinity into account. This could involve supporting men's possibilities to perform sexually as they age, which could involve retaining potency, but also to find alternative sexual practices to adapt to one's bodily ageing. In this the rights to information and education could play a central role. Sexual orientation should be brought into the picture since gay and bisexual men may, on the one hand, have invested heavily in masculinity throughout the life course to avoid homophobia and stigma but, on the other hand, also be more capable of negotiating normative gender.

A sexual rights perspective on older men should, moreover, challenge old-age negativity and ageist stereotypes of older men's sexualities, which may both involve the invisibility of older men as sexual subjects and depreciative images of "dirty old men". To what extent older men's sexualities are understood as desirable or problematic varies, however, depending on the privileges and vulnerabilities of different men. Existing research on the experiences of older men's sexuality, including the studies discussed previously, is primarily focused on community-dwelling relatively healthy men, rather than men in residential aged care facilities who are living with disabilities or chronic illnesses such as dementia. Studies of sexuality in these facilities suggest that male residents' sexual expressions are more often noted by staff than the sexual expressions of female residents, but also more often deemed problematic and a threat to a predominantly female workforce (Archibald 1998; Ward et al. 2005). Ward et al.'s study on caregivers' perceptions of sexuality and intimacy among residents with dementia suggests that non-heterosexual sexual expressions were often neglected, but Archibald's (1998) study on managers' responses also indicate that when male residents tried to fondle male staff, this was seen as more problematic than the fondling of female staff, as it challenged social norms on heterosexuality. Older men with disabilities, including men with dementia, could as such be understood as a group whose sexual rights are more threatened and who are at greater risk of facing degrading treatment (e.g. through libido suppressants). For older gay and bisexual men living in care homes, the combined effects of homophobia, ageism and negative attitudes to sexuality in dementia could in addition severely compromise sexual rights, health and well-being. More knowledge is also needed on how race and ethnicity intersect with the sexual rights of older men. Are, for example, sexual stereotypes of racialized men also influencing how they are understood as sexual subjects in later life?

As stated in the introduction to this chapter, the sexualities of older men are ambiguous. The concept of sexual dignity as central to older men's sense of self-worth may be a useful supplement to sexual rights terminology and help to clarify how men's sexualities are privileged in some contexts, yet acknowledge the vulnerability and obstacles that ageism, homophobia and normative masculinity impose on older men's sexual lives. We argue that the sexual rights of older men should include the liberty to express one's sexuality beyond negative ageist stereotyping but also beyond normative definitions of male sexuality that narrowly focus on sexual assertion and phallic sexuality.

References

Archibald, C. 1998, 'Sexuality, dementia and residential care: Managers' report and response', *Health and Social Care in the Community*, vol. 6, pp. 95–101.

Calasanti, T. & King, N. 2005, 'Firming the floppy penis: Class and gender relations in the lives of old men', *Men and Masculinities*, vol. 8, no. 1, pp. 3–23.

Calasanti, T., Slevin, K. & King, N. 2006, 'Ageism and feminism: From "Et Cetera" to Center', *NWSA Journal*, vol. 18, no. 1, pp. 13–30.

Cohler, B.J. 2004, 'Saturday night at the tubs: Age cohort and social life at the urban gay bath', in G. Herdt & B. deVries (eds.), *Gay and lesbian aging: Research and future directions*, Springer, New York.

Danoff, D.S. 1993, *Superpotency: How to get it, use it, and maintain it for a lifetime*, Warner Books, New York.

Fileborn, B., Thorpe, R., Hawkes, G., Minichiello, V., Pitts, M. & Dune, T. 2015, 'Sex, desire and pleasure: Considering the experiences of older Australian women', *Sexual and Relationship Therapy*, vol. 30, no. 1, pp. 117–30.

Fisher, L. 2010, *Sex, romance and relationships: 2009 AARP survey of midlife and older adults*, AARP, Washington DC, viewed 6 November 2016, http://assets.aarp.org/rgcenter/general/srr_09.pdf

Gledhill, S. & Schweitzer, R.D. 2014, 'Sexual desire, erectile dysfunction and the biomedicalization of sex in older heterosexual men', *Journal of Advanced Nursing*, vol. 70, no. 4, pp. 894–903.

Hennen, P. 2008, *Faeries, bears, and leathermen: Men in community queering the masculine*, University of Chicago Press, Chicago.

Horton, R. 2004, 'Rediscovering human dignity', *Lancet*, vol. 364, pp. 1081–85.

Hughes, J. 2011, 'Are older men taking sexuality as prescribed?: The implications of the competing influences on ageing male heterosexuality', *Australian Feminist Studies*, vol. 26, pp. 89–102.

Humphreys Laud 1970, *Tearoom Trade: A Study of Homosexual Encounters in Public Places,* New York: Aldine Publishing Company.

Kristiansen, H.W. 2004a, 'Kjærlighetskarusellen: Eldre homoseksuelle menns livsfortellinger og livsløp i Norge', PhD thesis, University of Oslo, Oslo, Norway.

Kristiansen, H.W. 2004b, 'Narrating past lives and present concerns: Older gay men in Norway', in G.H. Herdt & B. deVries (eds.), *Gay and lesbian aging: Research and future directions*, Springer, New York.

Kristiansen, H.W. 2008, *Masker og motstand. Diskré homoliv i Norge 1920–1970*, Unipub forlag, Oslo.

Kristiansen, H.W. 2013, 'Sexualitet och värdighet bland äldre homosexuella män i Norge', in J.A.S. Bromseth & A. Silverskog (eds.), *LHBT-personer och åldrande: nordiska perspektiv*, Studentlitteratur, Lund.

Loe, M. 2004, 'Sex and the senior woman: Pleasure and danger in the viagra era', *Sexualities*, vol. 7, no. 3, pp. 303–26.

Lottes, I.L. 2013, 'Sexual rights: Meanings, controversies, and sexual health promotion', *Journal of Sex Research*, vol. 50, no. 3–4, pp. 367–91.

Lyons, A., Croy, S., Barrett, C. & Whyte, C. 2015, 'Growing old as a gay man: How life has changed for the gay liberation generation', *Ageing and Society*, vol. 35, no 10, pp. 2229–50.

Marshall, B.L. 2006, 'The new virility: Viagra, male aging and sexual function', *Sexualities*, vol. 9, no. 3, pp. 345–62.

Marshall, B.L. 2010, 'Science, medicine and virility surveillance: "Sexy seniors" in the pharmaceutical imagination', *Sociology of Health & Illness*, vol. 32, no. 2, pp. 211–24.

Marshall, B.L. & Katz, S. 2002, 'Forever functional: Sexual fitness and the ageing male body', *Body & Society*, vol. 8, no. 4, pp. 43–70.

McCarthy, B., Farr, E. & McDonald, D. 2013, 'Couple sexuality after 60', *Journal of Family Psychotherapy*, vol. 24, no. 1, pp. 38–47.

Meadows, R.A.L. & Davidson, K. 2006, 'Maintaining manliness in later life: Hegemonic masculinities and emphasized femininities', in T. Calasanti & K. Slevin (eds.), *Age matters: Realigning feminist thinking*, Routledge, London.

Ménard, A.D., Kleinplatz, P.J., Rosen, L., Lawless, S., Paradis, N., Campbell, M. & Huber, J.D. 2015, 'Individual and relational contributors to optimal sexual experiences in older men and women', *Sexual and Relationship Therapy*, vol. 30, no. 1, pp. 78–93.

Mercer, J. 2014, 'Coming of age: Problematizing gay porn and the eroticized older man', *Journal of Gender Studies*, vol. 21, no. 3, pp. 313–26.

Oliffe, J. 2005, 'Constructions of masculinity following prostatectomy-induced impotence', *Social Science & Medicine*, vol. 60, no. 10, pp. 2249–59.

Potts, A., Gavey, N., Grace, V. & Vares, T. 2003, 'The downside of Viagra: Women's experiences and concerns', *Sociology of Health & Illness*, vol. 25, no. 7, pp. 697–719.

Potts, A., Grace, V., Vares, T. & Gavey, N. 2006, 'Sex for life?: Men's counter stories on "erectile dysfunction", male sexuality and ageing', *Sociology of Health and Illness*, vol. 28, no. 3, pp. 306–29.

Sandberg, L. 2011, 'Getting intimate: A feminist analysis of old age, masculinity & sexuality', PhD thesis, University of Linköping, Linköping, Sweden. [Available at: http://www.diva-portal.org/smash/get/diva2:408208/FULLTEXT01.pdf]

Sandberg, L. 2013, '"Just feeling a naked body close to you": Men, sexuality and intimacy in later life', *Sexualities*, vol. 16, pp. 261–82.

Sandberg, L. 2016, 'Inventions of hetero-sex in later life: Beyond dysfunction and the coital imperative', in N.L. Fischer & S. Seidman (eds.), *Introducing the new sexuality studies*, third edition, Routledge, London.

Slevin, K.F. & Linneman, T.J. 2010, 'Old gay men's bodies and masculinities', *Men and Masculinities*, vol. 12, pp. 483–507.

Smith, H.I. 2013, '"Momma's dead and daddy's on Viagra": Elder widowers, ED drugs, and new romantic relationships', in B DeFord & RB Gilbert (eds.), *Living, loving, and loss: The interplay of intimacy, sexuality, and grief*, Baywood Publishing Company, Amytiwille.

Suen, Y.T. 2015, 'To date or not to date, that is the question: Older single gay men's concerns about dating', *Sexual and Relationship Therapy*, vol. 30, no. 1, pp. 143–55.

Tiefer, L. 2004, 'Erectile dysfunction', in M.S. Kimmel & A. Aronson (eds.), *Men and masculinities: A social, cultural, and historical encyclopedia*, ABC-CLIO, Santa Barbara, CA.

Tiefer, L. 2006, 'The Viagra phenomenon', *Sexualities*, vol. 9, no. 3, pp. 273–94.

Wahler, J. & Gabbay, S.G. 1997, 'Gay male aging: A review of the literature', *Journal of Gay and Lesbian Social Services*, vol. 6, no. 3, pp. 1–20.

Ward, R., Vass, A. A., Aggarwal, N., Garfield, C., & Cybyk, B. 2005, 'A kiss is still a kiss? The construction of sexuality in dementia care', *Dementia,* vol. 4, no. 1, pp. 49–72.

Wentzell, E. 2011, 'Marketing silence, public health stigma and the discourse of risky gay Viagra use in the US', *Body & Society*, vol. 17, no. 4, pp. 105–25.

Wierzalis, E.A., Barret, B., Pope, M. & Rankins, M. 2006, 'Gay men and aging: Sex and intimacy', in D. Kimmel, T. Rose & S. David (eds.), *Lesbian, gay, bisexual, and transgender aging: Research and clinical perspectives*, Columbia University Press, New York.

5

THE HIDDEN SEXUALITIES OF OLDER LESBIANS AND BISEXUAL WOMEN

Sue Westwood and June Lowe

Introduction

In this chapter we consider how the sexualities of older lesbians and bisexual women are, for the most part, hidden from view, and reflect on the implications of this for sexual rights in later life (see Chapter 2 of this book). We explore how older lesbians' and bisexual women's invisibilisation is a creation of (in)equality, located at the intersections of ageism, sexism and heterosexism. We consider how these three discriminatory sites work with and through one another to render older lesbians and bisexual women invisible, which in turn denies and/or constrains their access to rights as ageing sexual beings.

We argue that the lack of recognition of older lesbians' and bisexual women's sexual rights can be understood in five pivotal ways: (1) an overarching breach of the right to equality and non-discrimination and of the right to access to justice, remedies and redress; (2) a breach of the right to information and of the right to education (both as older women and specific to their sexualities); (3) a breach of the right to the highest attainable health, including sexual health and the right to benefit from scientific progress and its application; (4) a breach of the right to enter, form and dissolve marriage and other similar types of relationships (which has particular significance in older age); and (5) a breach of three interlinked rights, related to older age in general, and care and support needs in particular, namely: (a) the right to freedom of thought, opinion and expression; (b) the right to freedom of association and peaceful assembly; and (c) the right to participation in public and political life. Our argument is that the invisibilisation of older lesbians' and bisexual women's sexualities needs to be understood not only as an *outcome* but also as an *ongoing process* of social marginalisation and exclusion. We conclude by suggesting how these processes might be remedied.

The chapter draws on the conceptual framework of intersectionality, which was first developed by Black feminist critical theorists (e.g. Crenshaw 1989), who sought to highlight how Black women experience racism differently from Black men and sexism differently from White women. Intersectionality has since developed into a wide-reaching paradigm (Taylor, Hines & Casey 2011), which offers a framework for understanding how different social divisions work with and through one another in inter-implicated ways to produce social inequalities. In the context of this chapter, the intersections that are of particular interest are those of age(ing), gender and sexuality.

Exploring sex and intimacy

Changing meanings of sex, sexualities and intimacy

Recent decades have seen dramatic changes in understandings of sex, sexuality and a growth in the rights of people with marginalised sexualities in many parts of the world (Stone & Weinberg 2015). What is understood by the term *sexuality* is itself open to debate (Weeks 2010), particularly in terms of whether it is an essential 'orientation', a behaviour, a politicised/strategic identity, a broader ethos, or mixtures of each. In terms of behaviour, much of the sexualities discourse is phallocentric and/or genital-centric, i.e. focussed on penetrative/genital sex (DeLamater & Plante 2015). This inherently invisibilises many women's sexualities, which may involve other forms of physical/non-physical intimacies, particularly for lesbians and bisexual women (Averett, Yoon & Jenkins 2012).

There is a growing recognition that, despite binary sexualities discourse (i.e. *either* heterosexual *or* lesbian/gay *or* bisexual), sexuality is actually far more fluid and complex. Since Kinsey's early work (Kinsey 1953), there has been an increasing appreciation of the overlap between same- and different-sex sexualities. Sexuality is, for many, contingent on social, cultural and historical context (Richardson 2000a), especially for women (Diamond 2008; Westwood 2013). Adrienne Rich's (1980) pivotal paper on compulsory heterosexuality highlighted how same-sex sexualities among women have been rendered not only prohibited but culturally *unthinkable*. While this attitude may be changing in some parts of the world, it still remains the case in many others, particularly where traditional religions inform cultural norms. The sexual/relational lives of older lesbians and bisexual women have traditionally been (and for many still are) navigated through and against this cultural censorship (Waite 2015; Traies 2016; Westwood 2016a).

Changing meanings of (older) lesbian sexualities

One of the problems with exploring (older) lesbians' lives is the issue of definitions and of 'never knowing, quite who is a lesbian' (Weston 2009, p. 136). Although good practice would suggest going for self-definition ('I am a lesbian' or 'I am lesbian'), this can exclude women with same-sex desires and/or in same-sex relationships who do not define themselves as lesbian (or bisexual) (Westwood 2013). Moreover, the word "lesbian" has multiple meanings for women who do identify with it (Traies

2016). Recent studies have demonstrated that the stories of older lesbians and/or non-labelling women in same-sex relationships reflect complex and diverse narratives of sexual fluidity and relational contingency. Westwood (2016a) conducted research with 60 older lesbian, gay and bisexual (LGB) people in the United Kingdom, exploring their experiences of later-life (in)equality. She concluded that their uneven access to resources, recognition and representation in later life is shaped by the intersection of age(ing) gender and sexuality, and by when and how a non-heterosexual identity/lifestyle emerged. She argued that this is especially the case for women, proposing that there are five different cohorts of older lesbian, bisexual and/or non-labelling women: 'Out Early'; 'Breaking Out'; 'Finding Out'; 'Late Performance'; and 'Lesbian by Choice' (p. 54). The 'Out Early' cohort refers to women in her study who had always identified as lesbian and said they had only ever had sexual relationships with women. For example, Moira, aged 75, "has always identified as lesbian and said she had only ever had sexual relationships with women: 'I'm a cradle lesbian. I was a lesbian at the age of three. . . . I fell in love at the age of nine for the first time'" (p. 54). The 'Breaking Out' cohort refers to women who were always aware of a same-sex sexuality but who went through an initial struggle with it before eventual resolution. For example, Diana, aged 69, came out in her twenties after wrestling with her sexuality:

> I was born in 1943. I knew there was something different about me. I had boyfriends. I was engaged, all that sort of thing. I didn't know there was anything other than heterosexuality, because that's all there was. But I knew I was different. . . . I had boyfriends while I was in the Navy. . . . I really believed that whatever my feelings were, they were just some sort of cross to bear . . . in my diaries. . . . I see my struggles at the time were my attractions to other women. I got friendly with a woman . . . it was normal, if you had a friend to stay, you shared a bed. And it happened, the second or third time we shared a bed, and it was the most natural thing in the world. And we thought we were the only ones [laughs].
>
> *(Westwood 2016a, p. 55)*

The 'Finding Out' cohort encompasses women who described growing self-awareness: 'I understand myself better now. . . . I see myself as lesbian now', Maureen, aged 62 (p. 56); 'and then I realised I preferred women', Rachel, aged 64 (p. 56); 'But then I fell in love with a woman, and then I knew what love was', May, aged 64 (p. 56). The 'Late Performance' cohort, by contrast, describes women who had lived heterosexual lives, with no awareness of sexual attraction towards women, before forming a sexual relationship with a woman late in life. They do not identify as lesbian/bisexual/gay, locating their sexualities in a relationship-contingent narrative. For example, Ellen was married to a man for 40 years before subsequently forming a relationship (and eventually civil partnership) with Tessa:

> I mean since I realised that I love Tessa, and love a woman, no-one could be more shocked than me, I can tell you . . . I've never fancied a woman in my

life. Present company excluded [said to Tessa] . . . I don't know if I am a lesbian, I really don't know. Am I a lesbian? All I know is I love Tessa, I love her to death . . . there's a very broad spectrum, isn't there? Because I lived as a heterosexual all my life, I didn't know as a child I was different, I didn't know as a young adult, middle adult, listening to lesbians talking, there's always been an innate knowledge, a recognition, even if it was denied. I've never had that recognition (Ellen, aged 64).

(Westwood 2016a, p. 57)

Lastly, the 'Lesbian by Choice' cohort refers to the – often unrecognised – political lesbians from the 1970s and 1980s, who 'gave up' men and chose a lesbian identity. For example, Jennifer assumed a lesbian identity and lifestyle, based on her radical feminist ideology, in the late 1970s:

I was a political lesbian. . . . I just made the choice to give up men. For all sorts of reasons, you know, it was the argument that I wanted someone who knew how to clean the toilet, and someone who didn't want me to cook for them, that sort of thing. . . . You see there are so many stories about 'I fell in love with a woman and there just was no choice', which is fine, it just wasn't what happened. I fell in love with lots of women and nothing happened, and I got off with lots of men, and I daresay I was in love with them, some of them, at various points. I mean this was the era when one did have lots of partners. And then I decided, no, I'm not going to have anything more to do with men. . . . So I gave up men. I didn't have any problems fancying women (Jennifer, aged 62, 'Lesbian by Choice').

(Westwood 2016a, p. 58)

This cohort analysis echoes Jane Traies' (2016) research with 400 older lesbians in the UK, where she found great diversity in the accounts of older lesbians. This complexity informs their invisibilisation: not only are they rendered invisible at the intersection of ageism, sexism and heterosexism, but they are also obscured in mono-constructions of ageing lesbianism, which fail to encompass the diversity and complexity of lesbian lives.

Changing meanings of (older) bisexual women's sexualities

Ageing bisexualities are marginalised in both generic ageing discourse, including about older women, and in lesbian, gay, bisexual and trans★[1] (LGBT★) ageing discourse. Rebecca Jones (2012) has written about the disappearing 'B' in LGBT★ discourse, wherein bisexuality rarely gets a mention beyond the acronym. This, of course, serves to obscure the lives, experiences, issues and concerns of all bisexual people, including older bisexual people and older bisexual women. There are again complexities of definition. Halperin (2009 pp. 453–4) has described a range of different ways of understanding bisexuality, in terms of sexual attraction, sexual behaviour, sexual desire and/or identity. Very often, bisexual women may find a greater sense of community with other bisexual women and men than with lesbians, partly because of different weightings given to the significance of gender in relation to sexuality. Although bisexuality is becoming increasingly accepted among young people in sexuality-liberal countries, ageing bisexual histories and lives remain far less well-recognised and/or understood (Jones 2016).

Sexual rights implications

In this section, we have highlighted how the lives of older lesbians and bisexual women are invisible, sometimes even to themselves. Without recognition of their sexualities, there can be no rights afforded to them and no formal rights claims made possible for them (Richardson 2000b).

Ageism, sexism and heterosexism

Older lesbians and bisexual women are under-represented in the literature about *both* older women (Cronin 2006; Westwood 2013, 2015) *and* about LGBT★ ageing (Barker 2004; Grossman 2008; Westwood 2013; Jones 2011; Traies 2016). This under-representation means that not only are their voices insufficiently well-heard but that also the (limited) stories of women's ageing are actually only stories of heterosexual women's ageing, and the stories of LGBT★ ageing tend to be stories that privilege the experiences of gay men (Averett & Jenkins 2012; Westwood 2017).

Older lesbians and bisexual women are located at the intersection of the 'organizing principles of power' (Calasanti & Slevin 2007, p. 10) of age, gender and sexuality and the combined and intertwined forces of ageism, sexism and heterosexism (Averett, Yoon & Jenkins 2012). Bisexual women are further marginalised by monosexism (i.e. the assumption that someone is *either* straight or lesbian/gay). Trans★ lesbians and trans★ bisexual women are also additionally affected by cisgenderism, that is, the assumption that people align with the sex/gender assigned to them at birth (Witten 2015).

Ageism (prejudice towards older people) and age discrimination (behaviours that treat older people differently because of their age) are powerful social forces (Bytheway 2005; Nelson 2004). In many cultures, older people are subject to profound cultural devaluation. With growing sociocultural pressures to age well or successfully, older people, especially 'younger' older people, are encouraged to mask the signs of ageing, physically and in terms of lifestyle. As long as they can remain youthful – sexy, active and engaged – they remain visible. However, this pushes those who are less able to age 'well' farther into the margins (Gilleard & Higgs 2010). This is further nuanced by gender: older women are subjected to cultural devaluation earlier and to a greater extent than are older men (Venn, Davidson & Arber 2011). Although 'successful ageing' is leading to increased representation of active sexuality among older women in popular culture, this is as long as they adhere to a certain version of respectable and 'age-appropriate' sexuality (Hinchliff 2014).

There have been mixed arguments as to whether older lesbians are subject to the same processes of invisibilisation as older heterosexual women (Slevin 2006; Averett, Yoon & Jenkins 2011): some authors have argued that because (some) older lesbians do not align themselves with heterosexual feminine norms, they are less susceptible to ageist exclusion associated with those norms; other authors have suggested that lesbians are ageing first and foremost as women and so are subject to the same marginalisations as heterosexual women. Older lesbians can also face ageism within lesbian communities (Copper 2015). For bisexual women, with their multiple, intersecting social positions, this can be even further complicated as they engage with 'non-normative' later lives (Jones 2011, 2012). What is most likely is that older lesbians and bisexual women are affected by the intersection of ageism, sexism and heterosexism in unique ways according to their particular circumstances, as they intersect with other social positions, including race/ethnicity (Woody 2015), class (Taylor 2009) and urban/rural spatial locations (Barefoot et al. 2015).

Ageing lesbian and bisexual women's lives

The shadow of the past

Social histories cast long shadows into the present. The formative years for young women and girls growing up in the first half of the 20th century were steeped in prevailing 19th-century ideas determining 'appropriate' (domestic, heterosexual) roles for women. Religious, medical and psychological ideologies were used to attack lesbian identities (Kennedy & Davis 2014). This wholesale social opprobrium set the conditions for hostility, denigration, and psychological, religious and physical violence (Waite 2015). Although in many countries lesbians escaped criminal sanctions that were applied to gay men, they were nonetheless subject to draconian 'cures', with homosexuality only being removed from the American *Diagnostic and Statistical Manual of Mental Disorders* (DSM) in 1973. Moral and medical stigma meant that women with children entering a lesbian relationship risked losing custody or access to them, and for many women today, the fracturing of family ties still has not healed.

Historic homophobia continues to shape many lesbians' sense of self and (lack of) safety. Older lesbians have experienced the pain of being socially outcast, considered sick, immoral, or an unfit mother, and have been at high risk of harassment and violence. Their only protection was often to make themselves invisible. In the face of pervasive persecution, living lesbian lives discreetly, or even in denial themselves, has been (and is) an important survival strategy, albeit one that perpetuates the myth of their own non-existence. This pattern of secrecy has important ramifications in the present time, contributing to social isolation and creating barriers to accessing appropriate care and support (Garner et al. 2014).

For an older bisexual woman, the experience of invisibility and minority stress can be amplified by a widespread lack of understanding of and/or respect for bisexuality (Dworkin 2006). In addition to the same invisibilising factors affecting lesbians, bisexual women's lives/identities are even more likely to be overlooked ('bi-erasure'), as perceptions of a bisexual woman's sexual identity are frequently linked to the gender of her current partner. Although bisexuality is, in recent times, attracting greater acceptance and may even be fashionable, an older bisexual woman is liable to have met with hostility by lesbians and unhelpful stereotypes in the broader community, being typecast as confused and/or amoral (Barker 2004). Unsurprisingly, many bisexual women may feel ambivalent about a bisexual label (Alarie & Gaudet 2013). An older bisexual woman can be disadvantaged by self-invisibilisation and alienated by double discrimination from both heterosexual and lesbian and gay worlds.

Ageing intimacies

Just as there are many diversities in lesbian and bisexual women's histories, so too there is great variation in their later-life relationship networks. For many older lesbians, particularly those with a life-long lesbian identity, peer networks, or 'families of choice', are central to their sense of self and well-being, and have been a crucial buffer against discrimination, mediating against marginality (Barrett et al. 2015). For others, particularly those previously in heterosexual relationships, with children and grandchildren, their biological families may have greater relative significance in their lives. Access to social capital in later life (Cronin & King 2014), particularly intergenerational support, is crucial to the well-being of older lesbians and bisexual women, and also informs if, when and/or how they are likely to require formal social support (Gabrielson 2011). Many older lesbians and bisexual women are carers to friends and/or family members, some of whom are older lesbians and bisexual women themselves (Traies 2015). Yet lesbian and bisexual carers are often under-recognised and under-supported by formal service providers (Manthorpe & Price 2006). For older lesbians and bisexual women, the legal recognition of same-sex partners, and of significant others, becomes a pressing later-life concern when facing issues relating to pensions, mental capacity, inheritance and funeral rights (Knauer 2010).

Health and social care and support needs

Many older lesbians and bisexual women remain resilient and in good health. However, a stressful life course and cumulative disadvantage has taken its toll on others (Hoy-Ellis & Fredriksen-Goldsen 2016). A range of studies suggest that older lesbians and bisexual women experience poorer physical and psychological health compared to older heterosexual women (e.g. Fredriksen-Goldsen et al. 2013). Barriers to accessing health care services, and in particular heteronormative providers (Neville et al. 2014), can inform a reluctance among older lesbians and bisexual women to access mainstream services for fear of ongoing discrimination. This in turn can have negative health outcomes. For example, lesbians face an increased risk of poor outcomes for breast and endometrial cancer, due to late presentation for diagnosis and treatment, based on fears of accessing potentially prejudiced and/or discriminatory mainstream services.

Much of health and social care provision is not geared up to the needs of older lesbians and bisexual women (Hughes 2007; Jones 2010; Grigorovich 2013), including those who are carers (Manthorpe & Price 2006; Hughes & Kentlyn, 2015). Providing culturally safe, inclusive services for older lesbians and bisexual women is imperative to ensure their human and sexual rights in terms of equal access to health and social care and quality care services for older people (Westwood et al. 2015). Key barriers to the provision of best practice care include these women's 'hidden' sexualities, both by their own self-guarding and by service providers' lack of regard or awareness, and heterosexist assumptions. Additionally, some service providers' staff and/or management may harbour ambivalence or hostility towards lesbian and bisexual sexualities, which can find expression in resistance to implementing change or reluctance to consider the need for transformative practices. Finally, pervasive heteronormativity presents a deep-rooted challenge to organisational change and inadvertently perpetuates exclusionary practices.

Dementia poses special concerns for lesbians and bisexual women, who are disproportionately affected compared with gay and bisexual men, primarily because dementia is age-related and women live longer than men (Westwood 2015). Disinhibition associated with dementia can place older lesbians/bisexual women at risk of disclosing their sexualities in ways that may compromise their or their partner's comfort or safety, especially if they were previously closeted about their sexuality (Price 2010). Being inadvertently 'outed' can expose individuals to prejudice, discrimination and heightened marginalisation (Duffy & Healy 2014).

Sexual rights implications

The lack of visibility of older lesbians and older bisexual women has a number of implications for their sexual rights, as follows:

1) *An overarching breach of the right to equality and non-discrimination and of the right to access to justice, remedies and redress*

Without recognition of older lesbians' and bisexual women's diverse and yet particular needs, those needs cannot be addressed in order to achieve equality. In terms of the three types of equality (Baker et al., 2016): (1) they cannot enjoy equal treatment when compared with older heterosexual women (because their specific needs, issues and concerns are not understood); (2) they cannot enjoy equal opportunity in terms of access to rights (because their rights are not defined); and, crucially, (3) they cannot have equality of outcome, in terms of engagement of rights (because their rights are not determined). It also then follows that without recognition of these rights, there can be no access to justice, remedies and redress, because there can be no rights claim-making, nor processes with which to challenge their breach. Moreover, (ageing) 'gay' and/or 'bisexual' rights that do not take gender into account fail to address how sexuality and gender intersect to produce inequality and marginalisation (Richardson 2000c).

2) *A breach of the right to information and of the right to education (both in general and sexuality-specific)*

Without recognition of older women's specific needs, wants, issues and concerns, older lesbians and bisexual women share with all older women the limited access to relevant information and education, including in relation to sexuality. Additionally, without recognition of older lesbians' and bisexual women's specific health and social care needs, there can be no targeted sexualities-specific information and education for (a) older lesbians and bisexual women themselves and (b) for LGBT★ groups and/or service providers for older people.

3) *A breach of the right to the highest attainable health, including sexual health and the right to benefit from scientific progress and its application*

The lack of recognition of the barriers facing lesbians and bisexual women of any age in terms of accessing women's health (including sexual health) care is compounded for older lesbians and bisexual women. They will have experienced a lifetime of this cumulative disadvantage and may be experiencing both its psychological and physical consequences. Older lesbians and bisexual women may be reluctant to engage with medical professionals by whom they have historically been pathologised and stigmatised. They may defer seeking a diagnosis, and therefore receive delayed treatments, and so experience poorer outcomes. They are therefore less likely to benefit from scientific progress/medical advances, because they are less likely to access them in timely ways.

4) *A breach of the right to enter, form and dissolve marriage and other similar types of relationships*

While in some countries same-sex marriage and/or other forms of partnership recognition now exist, this is not yet the case everywhere. Indeed, in some countries same-sex relationships are still illegal. Clearly, the lack of access to the same partnership rights as different-sex couples is a profound site of inequality. This is compounded in older age, when ageing partners may be concerned about pension and property rights, funeral rights and access to each other should one be hospitalised or placed in a care home. There is an enduring fear in such cases that biological family members may exclude the surviving/non-institutionalised partner, which, sadly, is known to still occur in those countries where partnership rights are lacking (Knauer 2010).

5) *Three interlinked rights: the right to freedom of thought, opinion and expression; the right to freedom of association and peaceful assembly; the right to participation in public and political life*

The minimal/lack of availability of safe public spaces for older lesbians and bisexual women in both LGBT★ circles and support spaces for older people (including health and social care services) means they have fewer opportunities to express their views, opinions, identities and histories than do younger LGBT★ people and older heterosexual women. These constraints also restrict their freedom of association (and peaceful assembly) and to participate in public and political life with other older lesbians and bisexual women (Westwood 2016b). While all older women are marginalised from active participation in public spaces in later life, at the intersection of ageism and sexism, this is compounded for older lesbians and bisexual women at the intersection of ageism and sexism with heterosexism, monosexism, homophobia and biphobia.

Possible remedies

Solutions to the marginalisation of older lesbians and bisexual women's sexual rights lie, in part, in the growing number of good examples of policies, practices and projects that render them visible and validate, support and empower them and the issues that concern them. They also lie in envisioning a new gender- and sexuality-informed imaginary in terms of conceptualising later life. In terms of policies, in some parts of the world (particularly Australia, Canada, the UK and USA), there is now a growing body of social policies and good practice guidelines for working well with older LGBT★ people in general and also particular members under the 'older LGBT★' umbrella, including older lesbians and bisexual women (Crameri et al. 2015; Westwood et al. 2015). In terms of practices, there is a growing number of specialist services (both community support and residential provision) for older LGBT★ people, within which there are sub-groups of support for older women and older bisexual people. There are a few (but only a very few) housing projects for older women internationally, with even fewer housing projects for older lesbians (Westwood, 2016b and 2017), and none specifically aimed at older bisexual people, let alone bisexual women. While not all older lesbians and bisexual women will want specialist services, the issue here is them having the choice between mainstream and specialist provision (Westwood 2016c). There are also a small number of older lesbian networks, notably, in the USA, Old Lesbians Organising for Change (OLOC)[2], a national network of lesbians over the age of 60 campaigning on behalf of old (sic) lesbians. There needs to be both more of all of the above in the countries where policies, good practice and projects do exist, and, of course, the creation of all of the above in those countries where they do not yet exist at all.

There needs to be a growing appreciation of sexual fluidity in older age, particularly for women, and increased recognition of the diversity of sexualities and sexual identities among older women in later life. Sexuality needs to be reconceptualised away from the phallocentric and genital-centric and more towards intimacy and affection, which better reflects the practices of many older women, particularly older lesbians, and older bisexual women in same-sex relationships. It needs to be understood as relational rather than as a (fixed) orientation, particularly for (older) women.

Conclusion

In this chapter we have outlined the historical and contemporary processes that invisibilise older lesbians and bisexual women. We have argued that their invisibilisation needs to be understood not only as an *outcome* but also as an *ongoing process* of social marginalisation and exclusion. With the increasing visibility of younger lesbians and bisexual women, and growing expectations of sexual rights, the need to achieve visibility and equity for older lesbians and bisexual women, within their own communities, LGBT★ communities and in the ageing community at large is not only a pressing concern, but one that is likely to become increasingly relevant in future decades.

Notes

1 Trans★ is an umbrella term that covers the gender identity spectrum, including (but not limited to) transgender, transsexual, transvestite, genderqueer, genderfluid, non-binary, genderless, agender, non-gendered, third gender, two-spirit and bigender (Tompkins 2014).
2 Old Lesbians Organising for Change, www.oloc.org

References

Alarie, M. & Gaudet, S. 2013, 'I don't know if she is bisexual or if she just wants to get attention': Analyzing the various mechanisms through which emerging adults invisibilize bisexuality, *Journal of Bisexuality*, vol *13*(2), pp. 191–214.

Averett, P. & Jenkins, C. 2012, Review of the literature on older lesbians: Implications for education, practice, and research, *Journal of Applied Gerontology*, vol *31*(4), pp. 537–561.

Averett, P., Yoon, I. & Jenkins, C. L. 2011, Older lesbians: Experiences of aging, discrimination and resilience, *Journal of Women & Aging*, vol *23*(3), pp. 216–232.

Averett, P., Yoon, I. and Jenkins, C.L., 2012, Older lesbian sexuality: Identity, sexual behavior, and the impact of aging, *Journal of Sex Research*, *49*(5), pp. 495–507.

Baker, J., Lynch, K., Cantillon, S. and Walsh, J. 2016, *Equality: From theory to action*, Springer, New York.

Barefoot, K. N., Rickard, A., Smalley, K. B. & Warren, J. C. 2015, Rural lesbians: Unique challenges and implications for mental health providers, *Journal of Rural Mental Health*, vol *39*(1), p. 22.

Barker, J. C. 2004, Lesbian ageing: An agenda for social research, in G. Herdt & B. De Vries (eds.) *Gay and lesbian ageing: Research and future directions*, Springer, New York, pp. 29–72.

Barrett, C., Whyte, C., Comfort, J., Lyons A. & Crameri P. 2015, Social connection, relationships and older lesbian and gay people, *Sexual and Relationship Therapy*, vol *30*(1), pp. 131–142.

Bytheway, B. 2005, Ageism and age categorization, *Journal of Social Issues*, vol *61*(2), pp. 361–374.

Calasanti, T. & Slevin, K. (eds.) 2007, *Age matters: Realigning feminist thinking*, Routledge, New York.

Copper, B. 2015, Ageism in the lesbian community, *Journal of Lesbian Studies*, vol *19*(1), pp. 7–12.

Crameri, P., Barrett, C., Latham, J. R. & Whyte, C., 2015, It is more than sex and clothes: Culturally safe services for older lesbian, gay, bisexual, transgender and intersex people, *Australasian Journal on Ageing*, vol *34*(S2), pp. 21–25.

Crenshaw, K. 1989, Demarginalizing the intersection of race and sex: A black feminist critique of antidiscrimination doctrine, feminist theory and antiracist politics, *University of Chicago Legal Forum*, pp. 139–167.

Cronin, A. 2006, Sexuality in gerontology: A heteronormative presence, a queer absence, in S. O. Daatland & S. Biggs (eds.) *Ageing and diversity: Multiple pathways & cultural migrations*, Policy Press, New York, pp. 107–122.

Cronin, A. & King, A. 2014, Older lesbian, gay and bisexual (LGB) adults and social capital, *Ageing and Society*, vol *34*(2), pp. 258–279, doi: 10.1017/S0144686£12000955.

DeLamater, J. & Plante, R. F. (eds.) 2015, *Handbook of the sociology of sexualities*, Springer, New York.

Diamond, L. M. 2008, *Sexual fluidity: Understanding women's love and desire*, Harvard University Press, Cambridge, MA.

Duffy, F. & Healy, J. P. 2014, A social work practice reflection on issues arising for LGBTI older people interfacing with health and residential care: Rights, decision making and end-of-life care, *Social Work in Health Care*, vol *53*(6), pp. 568–583.

Dworkin, S. H. 2006, The ageing bisexual: The invisible of the invisible minority, in D. Kimmel, T. Rose & S. David (eds.) *Lesbian, gay, bisexual and transgender aging*, Columbia University Press, New York, pp. 36–52.

Fredriksen-Goldsen, K. I., Emlet, C. A., Kim, H. J., Muraco, A., Erosheva, E. A., Goldsen, J. & Hoy-Ellis, C. P. 2013, The physical and mental health of lesbian, gay male, and bisexual (LGB) older adults: The role of key health indicators and risk and protective factors, *The Gerontologist*, vol *53*(4), pp. 664–675.

Gabrielson, M. L. 2011, 'We have to create family': Aging support issues and needs among older lesbians, *Journal of Gay & Lesbian Social Services*, vol *23*(3), pp. 322–334.

Garner, J. D., Clunis, D. M., Freeman, P. A., Nystrom, N. M. & Fredriksen-Goldsen, K. I. 2014, *Lives of lesbian elders: Looking back, looking forward*, Routledge, New York.

Gilleard, C. & Higgs, P. 2010, Aging without agency: Theorizing the fourth age, *Aging & Mental Health*, vol *14*(2), pp. 121–128.

Grigorovich, A. 2013, Long-term care for older lesbian and bisexual women: An analysis of current research and policy, *Social Work in Public Health*, vol *28*(6), pp. 596–606.

Grossman, A. 2008, Conducting research among older lesbian, gay and bisexual adults, *Journal of Gay and Lesbian Social Services*, vol *20*, pp. 51–67.

Halperin, D. M. 2009, Thirteen ways of looking at a bisexual, *Journal of Bisexuality*, vol *9*(3–4), pp. 451–455.

Hinchliff, S. 2014, Sexing-up the midlife woman: Cultural representations of ageing, femininity, and the sexy body, in I. Whelehan & J. Gwynne (eds.) *Ageing, popular culture and contemporary feminism: Harleys and hormones*, Palgrave, Basingstoke, UK, pp. 63–77.

Hoy-Ellis, C.P. & Fredriksen-Goldsen, K.I. 2016, Lesbian, gay, & bisexual older adults: Linking internal minority stressors, chronic health conditions, and depression, *Aging & Mental Health*, *20*(11), pp.1119–1130.

Hughes, M. 2007, Older lesbians and gays accessing health and aged-care services, *Australian Social Work*, vol *60*(2), pp. 197–209.

Hughes, M. & Kentlyn, S. 2015, Older lesbians and work in the Australian health and aged care sector, *Journal of Lesbian Studies*, vol *19*(1), pp. 62–72.

Jones, R. 2010, Troubles with bisexuality in health and social care, in R. Jones & R. Ward (eds.) *LGBT issues: Looking beyond categories*, Dunedin, Edinburgh, pp. 42–55.

Jones, R. 2011, Imagining bisexual futures: Positive, non-normative later life, *Journal of Bisexuality*, vol *11*(2–3), pp. 245–270.

Jones, R. 2012, Imagining the unimaginable: Bisexual roadmaps for ageing, in R. Ward, I. Rivers & M. Sutherland (eds.) *Lesbian, gay, bisexual and transgender ageing: Biographical approaches for inclusive care and support*, Jessica Kingsley Press, London, pp. 21–38.

Jones, R. 2016, Aging and bisexuality, in A. E. Goldberg (ed.) *The Sage encyclopedia of LGBTQ studies*, Sage, New York, pp. 57–61.

Kennedy, E. L. & Davis, M. D. 2014, *Boots of leather, slippers of gold: The history of a lesbian community*, Routledge, New York.

Kinsey, A. C., Pomeroy, W. B., Martin, C. E., & Gebhard, P. H. 1953, *Sexual behavior in the human female*, Indiana University Press, Bloomington, IN.

Knauer, N. J. 2010, Gay and lesbian elders: Estate planning and end-of-life decision making, *Florida Coastal Law Review*, vol *11*, pp. 2011–2016.

Manthorpe, J. & Price, E. 2006, Lesbian carers: Personal issues and policy responses, *Social Policy and Society*, vol *5*(1), pp. 15–26.

Nelson, T.D. (ed.), 2004, *Ageism: Stereotyping and prejudice against older persons*, MIT Press, Boston, MA.

Neville, S., Adams, J., Bellamy, G., Boyd, M. & George, N. 2014, Perceptions towards lesbian, gay and bisexual people in residential care facilities: A qualitative study, *International Journal of Older People Nursing*, vol *10*, pp. 73–81.

Price, E. 2010, Coming out to care: Gay and lesbian carers' experiences of dementia services, *Health & Social Care in the Community*, vol *18*(2), pp. 160–168.

Rich, A. 1980, Compulsory heterosexuality and lesbian existence, *Signs*, vol *5*(4), pp. 631–660.

Richardson, D. 2000a, *Rethinking sexuality*, Sage, London.

Richardson, D. 2000b, Constructing sexual citizenship: Theorising sexual rights, *Critical Social Policy*, vol *61*(4), pp. 105–135.

Richardson, D. 2000c, Claiming citizenship? Sexuality, citizenship and lesbian/feminist theory, *Sexualities*, vol *3*(2), pp. 255–272.

Slevin, K. 2006, The embodied experiences of old lesbians, in T. Calasanti & K. Slevin (eds.) *Age matters: Realigning feminist thinking*, Routledge, New York, pp. 247–268.

Stone, A. L. & Weinberg, J. D. 2015, Sexualities and social movements: Three decades of sex and social change, in J. DeLamater & R. F. Plante (eds.) *Handbook of the sociology of sexualities*, Springer, New York, pp. 453–465.

Taylor, Y. 2009, Complexities and complications: Intersections of class and sexuality, *Journal of Lesbian Studies*, vol *13*(2), pp. 189–203.

Taylor, Y., Hines, S. & Casey, M. 2011, Introduction, in Y. Taylor, S. Hines & M. E. Casey (eds.) *Theorizing intersectionality and sexuality*, Palgrave Macmillian, Basingstoke, pp. 1–12.

Tompkins, A. 2014, Asterisk, *TSQ: Transgender Studies Quarterly*, vol *1*(1–2), pp. 26–27.

Traies, J. 2015, Old lesbians in the UK: Community and friendship, *Journal of Lesbian Studies*, vol *19*(1), pp. 35–49.

Traies, J. 2016, *The lives of older lesbians: Sexuality, identity and the life course*, Springer, New York.

Venn, S., Davidson, K. & Arber, S. 2011, Gender and aging, in R. A. Settersten (ed.) *Handbook of sociology of aging*, Springer, New York, pp. 71–81.

Waite, H. 2015, Old lesbians: Gendered histories and persistent challenges, *Australian Journal on Ageing*, vol *34*(2), pp. 8–13.

Weeks, J. 2010, *Sexuality*, third edition, Routledge, London.

Weston, K. 2009, The lady vanishes: On never knowing, quite, who is a lesbian, *Journal of Lesbian Studies*, vol *13*(2), pp. 136–148.

Westwood, S. 2013, Researching older lesbians: Problems and partial solutions, *Journal of Lesbian Studies*, vol *17*(3–4), pp. 380–392.

Westwood, S. 2015, Dementia, women and sexuality: How the intersection of ageing, gender and sexuality magnify dementia concerns among older lesbian and bisexual women, *Dementia: The International Journal of Social Research and Practice*, doi: 1471301214564446.

Westwood, S. 2016a, *Ageing, gender and sexuality: Equality in later life*, Routledge, Abingdon.

Westwood, S. 2016b, LGBT★ ageing in the UK: Spatial inequalities in older age housing/care provision, *Journal of Poverty and Social Justice*, vol *24*(1), pp. 63–76.

Westwood, S. 2016c, 'We see it as being heterosexualised, being put into a care home': Gender, sexuality and housing/care preferences among older LGB individuals in the UK, *Health and Social Care in the Community*, doi: 10.1111/hsc.12265 http://onlinelibrary.wiley.com/doi/10.1111/hsc.12265/abstract

Westwood, S. 2017, Gender and older LGBT★ housing discourse: the marginalised voices of older lesbians, gay and bisexual women. *Housing, Care and Support*, 20.

Westwood, S., King, A., Almack, K. & Suen, Y.-T. 2015, Good practice in health and social care provision for older LGBT people, in J. Fish & K. Karban (eds.) *Social work and lesbian, gay, bisexual and trans health inequalities: International perspectives*, Policy Press, Bristol, pp. 145–159.

Witten, T. M. 2015, Elder transgender lesbians: Exploring the intersection of age, lesbian sexual identity, and transgender identity, *Journal of Lesbian Studies*, vol *19*(1), pp. 73–89.

Woody, I. 2015, Lift every voice: Voices of African-American lesbian elders, *Journal of Lesbian Studies*, vol *19*(1), pp. 50–58.

6

TRANSGENDER OLDER PEOPLE

At sea far from the sexual rights shore

Loree Cook-Daniels and Michael Munson

Introduction

In modern Western culture, the lives of transgender older people are rife with discrimination, stigma, and violence; circumscribed; regulated; and even, sometimes, denied outright. Given how much injustice they experience and how much they are denied well-established basic human rights, asserting their sexual rights is a nearly insurmountable challenge.

This chapter explores how the circumstances in which transgender older people live complicate or even preclude assertion of each of the 15 sexual rights outlined in Chapter 2. It will discuss how each right is uniquely constrained by the circumstances in which transgender older people are forced to exist. Because research on transgender older people is largely non-existent, in many instances the discussion will focus on what is known about transgender adults of all ages. Where transgender aging research does exist, it has largely been based on U.S. and certain European populations, limiting applicability.

The cultural context

Many present-day as well as past cultures have more than two genders and/or acknowledge that individuals may be a gender different from what their bodily configuration might suggest (Feinberg 1996; Roscoe 1998). For many centuries in modern Western cultures, however, legally as well as socially there are only two ("binary") genders, each permanently associated with a particular genital configuration ("immutable"). Because of this codified belief, for many generations virtually all transgender individuals have either done their best to suppress their gender identity or have left their homes and families and turned up elsewhere in a different gender, never revealing their history or bodies, sometimes even to spouses (Stryker

2008). These transgender pioneers are typically known now only because their status was literally revealed in death.

Some living Western transgender elders still fall into that latter, hidden, category. With or without medical help, legal document changes, or other assistance, these individuals "transitioned" (began living as another gender) decades ago, and have lived quietly ever since simply as a man or a woman. Many have actively avoided contact with other transgender people or even lesbian, gay, bisexual and transgender (LGBT) communities, sometimes because they felt safer from possible suspicions and social disparagements that way. Obviously, this segment of transgender elders is by definition unstudied and unserved. They typically avoid even routine health care (to avoid having their transgender history come to light), and would certainly never reveal their histories to a researcher. We will likely never know much about them.

The larger segment of living Western transgender elders spent many decades fighting or trying to change their gender identity. These individuals often chose hyper-masculine or hyper-feminine professions or roles in attempts to suppress their feelings. For example, despite the fact that transgender people were formally banned from serving in the U.S. military until 2016, transgender individuals in the U.S. are twice as likely to be military veterans as are their non-transgender peers (Harrison-Quintana & Herman 2013).

At this point it is clear that many, if not most, such individuals failed in their suppression efforts. Once the internet's establishment gave these individuals a way to find a name for their feelings and learn another way of coping – by transitioning to live as the other gender – many of them found continued suppression impossible. Thus, many transgender people who are currently age 65 or older only "transitioned" relatively late in life. Indeed, an age-based analysis of the 2011 U.S. "National Transgender Discrimination Study" found that 97% of their 65+ respondents had transitioned at age 55 or later (National Center for Transgender Equality 2011).

One of the results of the unique historical trends that shaped today's cohort of transgender elders is that our knowledge of their lives is extremely limited. Many remain "invisible" to researchers, as being transgender is not an identity they claim or make public. Those who are public spent most of their lives trying to suppress their gender, only relatively recently admitting their identity and/or taking steps to live in their authentic gender. Therefore, there has been little time to gather data on them either. Of necessity, then, much of this discussion will focus on transgender adults in general – about whom we know more – than it will on transgender elders.

Sexual rights in a transgender elder context

Equality and non-discrimination (#1)

> Older people are entitled to enjoy all sexual rights set out in this declaration without distinction of any kind, such as race, ethnicity, color, gender, sex, language, religion, political or other opinion, national or social origin, place of residence, property, birth, disability, age, nationality, marital or

family status, sexual orientation, gender identity and expression, health status, economic and social situation and other status.

The first barrier to sexual rights for transgender elders is far, far higher than it is for the other elders in this book: they have to prove their very existence. Here are three recent, widely publicized medical doctors' opinions on the topic:

> Dr. Joseph Berger has issued a statement saying that from a medical and scientific perspective there is no such thing as a 'transgendered' person.
> *(Lifesitenews.com 2013)*

> Dr. Keith Ablow . . . [says] he's not convinced that being transgender is a real sexual identity.
> *(Feldman 2014)*

> Dr. Paul R. McHugh . . . [says] sex change is 'biologically impossible'.
> *(Chapman 2016)*

Transgender critics say that being transgender – having a gender identity and/or living as a gender that does not match what one was assumed to be at birth – is to have a "mental disorder" (Dr. McHugh), to be the victim of "delusions, psychosis or emotional unhappiness" (Dr. Berger), and is "profoundly destructive, psychologically" to not just trans people themselves, but "to all students" exposed to the idea that sex is not immutable (Dr. Ablow). If your very identity is deemed not "real" – let alone "profoundly destructive" to young children – it's highly unlikely that your sexual rights will be honored.

Another part of the problem is that gender identity and sexuality are widely confused with each other. Many people believe that transgender women are actually men who are attracted to other men but who are so resistant to the label "gay" that they would rather live as a woman. This construct is widely refuted by lesbian, gay, bisexual, and transgender (LGBT) activists, who teach that sexual orientation and gender identity are two completely separate variables: one is about the gender(s) you are attracted to and the other is your internal sense of self. One transgender elder answered a survey question asking how their sexuality interacts with a transgender history/identity this way:

> Laughing . . . it doesn't. Trans is an umbrella term that goes, and goes, and goes . . . on for ever, ever, ever, ever, ever, ever ever. Who I am is not a medical condition. Does your root canal affect your sexuality and identity?

On the other hand, the majority of trans elders that FORGE surveyed said their (or their partner's) (trans)gender identity had "completely" (22%) or "somewhat" shaped their sexuality (48%) (Cook-Daniels & Munson 2010). Only 29% asserted that their own or their partner's transgender identity had had "no effect" on their sexuality.

Speaking of those partners brings us to another complication in the discussion of the sexual rights of transgender elders: most sexual partners of transgender people are not themselves transgender. Yet they are clearly literal partners in transgender elders' sexuality. Moreover, they are often subjected to the same social approbation and discrimination as are their transgender partners. The International Transgender Day of Remembrance list of transgender people murdered because of their gender identity includes several non-transgender partners who were killed alongside their loved ones. The 2011 U.S. National Transgender Discrimination Study found that 14% of the partners of transgender people had experienced job discrimination because of their partner's gender identity, a statistic that doubled to 28% if the transgender person also experienced job discrimination (Grant et al. 2011).

Life, liberty and security (#2)

> Older people have the right to life, liberty and security that cannot be arbitrarily threatened, limited or taken away for reasons related to sexuality. These include sexual orientation, consensual sexual behavior and practices, gender identity and expression or because of accessing or providing services related to sexual and reproductive health.

Between 2008 and 2015, the murders of 2,016 transgender people in 65 countries were recorded (Balzar 2016). Those who were particularly likely to be murdered were transgender people who engage in sex work to survive. Transgender Europe reports that among those murder victims whose profession was known, 65% were sex workers (Balzar 2016).

Commercial sex work is strongly associated with transgender individuals in both reality and stereotype. Discrimination, prejudice and abuse pave the pathway to sex work, and transgender individuals are too often forced onto that pathway as soon as they are identified as, or declare themselves to be, gender non-conforming (which could be as early as preschool). Parental abuse and rejection, school-based bullying, and "guidance" from teachers and other adults to make the child conform to their society's gender norms can create pressures to leave school and/or the family home before education has been completed and full life skills developed. Dropping out of school and becoming homeless both raise adolescents' risks of using sex work to survive, a tendency that can be reinforced when more traditional employers refuse to hire or practice discrimination against transgender applicants and employees. Sex workers face even more limited future employment options if they ever obtain a criminal record because their work is deemed illegal.

The world's largest survey of transgender people (James et al. 2016) found that 12% of transgender individuals in the U.S. – including transgender men as well as transgender women – had engaged in sex work at some point in their lifetime. In countries where sex work is illegal, risk of loss of liberty (i.e. incarceration) is obviously much higher for those who are both transgender and surviving through sex work. In addition, many transgender people who are not sex workers are nevertheless treated as such, particularly by law enforcement officers who assume that all transgender women, especially if they are women of color, are prostitutes.

As a result, incarceration rates among transgender individuals are extremely high – 16% of trans people in the U.S. have been to jail or prison for any reason, compared to 2.7% of the general U.S. population – a figure that rises exponentially (up to 47%) for trans women of color (Grant et al. 2011).

Discrimination and harassment both in school and in the workplace is the cause of many transgender individuals entering into sex work. It is important to note that while the risk of both being murdered and the percentage of people doing sex work are generally much higher for younger adults, elders are not exempt. One trans elder told the authors:

> I prostitute myself at age 55 because even though I'm a [post-operative trans-sexual] and passable [as a woman], no one passes 100% of the time. NO ONE. Job discrimination is bad because you're stuck with fellow employees 8 hours a day, 40 hours a week. That much harassment is bad for one's mental health.
> *(Cook-Daniels & Munson 2010)*

Autonomy and bodily integrity (#3)

> *Older people have the right to control and decide freely on matters related to their sexuality and their body. This includes the choices of sexual behaviours, practices, partners and relationships with due regard to the rights of others. Free and informed decision-making requires free and informed consent prior to any sexually-related testing, interventions, therapies, surgeries or research.*

Transgender elders by definition face many challenges to their autonomy and bodily integrity. Although not all transgender people want to use hormones and/or have surgery to alter their bodies, many do. Whether they can access these medical services depends on political will (where medicine is socialized or legislated), insurance coverage decisions (for those transgender individuals who have insurance), and individual health care providers' knowledge, training, and personal attitudes. As an example, in the United States, transgender individuals' access to hormones and surgeries was widely blocked by federal health programs and by private insurance companies; only under the Obama Administration did these prohibitions begin to fall.

Those who "oppose" transgender people also use variations of the notion of "free and informed consent" to try to limit transgender individuals' autonomy. The original 1981 Medicare prohibition against gender confirmation surgery (GCS; one or more surgeries to bring a person's body more in line with their gender identity) stemmed from an essay written by notorious anti-transgender feminist activist Janice Raymond, who penned a document that U.S. government officials used to state that the surgeries are "controversial" and "experimental," and that there is a "lack of well controlled, long-term studies of the safety and effectiveness of the surgical procedures" and "a high rate of serious complications of these surgical procedures" (Williams 2014).

Nearly 30 years and tens of thousands of surgeries later, there are still critics who seek to limit the medical rights of transgender individuals by arguing that "informed consent" is irrelevant because the surgery does not actually improve transgender people's lives. Dr. Paul McHugh, who participated in gender confirmation surgeries at the U.S.'s Johns Hopkins University before experiencing a change of heart, points to a 30-year study of transgender individuals who did and did not have GCS (McHugh 2016). He notes that most of those who had surgery were "satisfied" with the results, but he finds it far more significant that "their subsequent psycho-social adjustments were no better than those who didn't have the surgery" (McHugh 2016). Apparently surgery on a usually hidden part of the body failed to cure the kinds of social discrimination and harassment that are more typically viewed as primary influences on the "psycho-social adjustments" of stigmatized minorities.

Being denied medical care one views as critical to one's physical and mental health has far-reaching repercussions for transgender older people. Such denials, particularly when accompanied by widespread public condemnation and ridicule over one's very identity, tend to erode transgender older persons' ability and willingness to advocate for their other rights, including those related to sexual behaviors.

Degrading treatment or punishment (#4)

> Older people have the right to be free from torture and cruel, inhuman or degrading treatment or punishment related to sexuality including that which is perpetrated for reasons related to someone's sex, gender, sexual orientation, gender identity and expression and bodily diversity.

The lives of transgender people are so far from being "free from torture and cruel, inhuman or degrading treatment or punishment" that one key study (Grant et al. 2011, p. 2) opened with this paragraph:

> Transgender and gender non-conforming people face injustice at every turn: in childhood homes, in school systems that promise to shelter and educate, in harsh and exclusionary workplaces, at the grocery store, the hotel front desk, in doctors' offices and emergency rooms, before judges and at the hands of landlords, police officers, health care workers and other service providers.

Several years later, a second survey drew 27,715 transgender respondents who affirmed that while some things were improving, degrading treatment or punishment was still pervasive (James et al. 2016). Reporting only on incidents from the year prior to the survey, discrimination due to gender identity or expression tallies included:

- 58% of those interacting with law enforcement reported experiencing some form of mistreatment by officers.
- 46% had experienced verbal harassment in the past year.
- 33% of those who had sought health care in the past year had experienced at least one negative experience in a health care setting.
- 31% had experienced some type of mistreatment in a place of public accommodation (restaurant, government office, etc.).
- 30% of employed respondents reported having been fired, denied a promotion, or experiencing some other form of workplace mistreatment.
- 23% had experienced some form of housing discrimination.
- 9% had been denied access to a restroom.

Obviously, transgender older adults experience overwhelming rates of degradation and punishment in many areas of their public and private lives. These experiences clearly diminish transgender older people's willingness to access other services and supports that will enable them to exercise their sexual rights. The same study quoted above found that nearly one-quarter (23%) of transgender respondents had skipped needed health care in the past year alone due to fear they would be mistreated in the health care setting.

Violence and coercion (#5)

> Everyone shall be free from sexuality related violence and coercion including: rape, sexual abuse, sexual harassment, bullying, sexual exploitation, and violence committed because of real or perceived sexual practices, sexual orientation, gender identity and expression and bodily diversity.

Along with degrading treatment, transgender people face staggering levels of violence and coercion. The *United States Transgender Survey* (Grant et al. 2011) documented some of the following statistics:

- 54% had experienced some form of intimate partner violence.
- 47% had been sexually assaulted at least once.
- 35% had experienced physical violence by an intimate partner.
- 10% had been sexually assaulted in the year prior to the survey.
- 10% had experienced a family member's violence toward them because of their gender identity.
- 9% had been physically attacked in the year prior to the survey.

Transgender people who experience violence often have a hard time accessing assistance. As noted above, law enforcement officers are frequently abusive to transgender victims. In the U.S. and Canada, as well as other countries, the service systems set up to help victims of domestic and sexual violence are typically focused solely on non-transgender female victims. Both transgender men and transgender women report being denied equal treatment or service, verbally harassed, or physically attacked by staff of domestic violence shelters and programs or rape crisis centers who knew or suspected they were transgender. That happened to 22% of those who tried to access such services in the past year; twice as many transgender people who needed such services did not even seek them due to fear of mistreatment (Grant et al. 2011).

An additional barrier facing half of the transgender community is the widespread myth that sexual assault and intimate partner violence are "gender-based violence," or violence perpetrated by men against women. In fact, the authors' own studies have found that transgender men are even more likely to experience these forms of violence than are transgender women (Cook-Daniels & Munson 2016). In an effort to defend the myth that "male privilege" protects transgender men from sexual and intimate partner violence, some transgender activists have actively denigrated transgender men who disclose their abuse experience, charging that such discussions "take attention away from where it belongs," typically identified as transgender women of color (Cook-Daniels 2016).

Privacy (#6)

Older people have the right to privacy related to sexuality, sexual life and choices regarding their own body and consensual sexual relations and practices without arbitrary interferences and intrusion. This includes the right to control the disclosure of sexuality related personal information to others.

One of the most common complaints that transgender individuals of all ages have is that many people – including service providers – believe that typical privacy norms become totally optional when talking with someone who is transgender. Thus, it is common for transgender people to be asked about their genitals, their medical history, and even "how you have sex." Particularly when they come from health care or other service providers, these questions force transgender patients and clients to weigh whether asserting their privacy rights is more important than obtaining the services they are seeking.

More systemically, transgender people are deprived of their privacy by laws and policies that make it difficult, if not impossible, to change their identification documents to reflect a new name and correct gender identity, thus forcing them to produce "incongruent" identification that effectively discloses their transgender status or history.

Health, pleasurable and safe sexual experiences (#7)

Older people have the right to the highest attainable level of health and wellbeing in relation to sexuality, including the possibility of pleasurable, satisfying and safe sexual experiences. This requires the availability, accessibility, acceptability of quality health services and access to the conditions that influence and determine health including sexual health.

Access to quality health services is an ongoing problem for transgender elders. Health care professionals typically receive little or no training on the health needs of transgender people, and many carry into their practices high levels of ignorance and/or bias that result in poor care. In a large recent U.S. survey (James et al. 2016), 24% of transgender people who had received health care in the past year had to educate their own doctors about transgender health issues. Fifteen percent (15%) were asked inappropriate, unrelated questions about their body or sexuality, and 9% were refused health care outright. Transgender patients also reported that in the last year in health care providers' offices they had experienced verbal harassment, physical attack, and even sexual assault. These statistics relate to general health care as well as transition-related healthcare; the quality of sexual health services for transgender elders is unknown but, based on more basic care experiences, likely far from adequate.

Scientific progress and its application (#8)

Older people have the right to enjoy the benefits of scientific progress and its application in relation to sexuality and sexual health.

Prejudice and discrimination against stigmatized minorities like transgender people seem quite immune to scientific progress. In the U.S., the most recent political debates around the rights of transgender people have focused on the "danger" transgender people pose to other users of public restrooms. Even the more nuanced arguments that explain that it is not transgender people themselves who are dangerous, but men falsely stating they are transgender, fail to take into account decades' worth of evidence that the vast majority of both male and female rapists choose as victims people they have relationships with as opposed to selecting a stranger at random in public (RAINN n.d.). Scientific evidence is absolutely clear: people who are truly concerned with reducing sexual assaults should be focusing their efforts on processing existing rape kits and educating adults on the ways in which pedophiles meet and "groom" their young victims (Cook-Daniels 2016). Instead, creating and advertising a false linkage between transgender people and rapists creates an environment in which all aspects of transgender elders' lives – including but certainly not limited to sexuality and sexual health – are negatively affected.

Opposition to settled scientific evidence on transgender older persons, particularly when codified into restrictive laws, has tremendously negative effects. For example, the *U.S. Transgender Survey* found the following practical implications of the fears people have about transgender people in public restrooms. In the past year alone,

- 24% had been questioned or challenged over their public restroom use.
- 9% had been denied access to a public restroom.
- 12% had been verbally attacked, physically attacked, or sexually assaulted when accessing a public restroom.

- 59% had avoided using a public restroom to try to avoid being harassed there.
- 32% limited the amount they ate or drank to lessen their need to use a public restroom.
- 8% reported having had a urinary tract infection, kidney infection, or other kidney-related problem as a result of avoiding public restrooms (James et al. 2016).

Information provision (#9)

> Older people have the right to access to scientifically accurate and understandable information related to sexuality, sexual health and sexual rights through diverse sources. Such information should not be arbitrarily censored, withheld or intentionally misrepresented.

There is virtually no research on the sexuality of transgender elders, making dissemination of scientifically accurate and understandable sexuality information literally impossible. Often even basic information is lacking; the authors once consulted with a long-standing HIV-prevention program focused solely on transgender people and realized mid-meeting that the leaders had no idea that hormone use could alter physical functioning to a point where traditional safer sex practices simply do not work.

Transgender people also suffer from experts' misconceptions. An online video by a transgender man illustrates how stereotypes about the ways in which HIV can be transmitted not only prevented him from getting the care he needed, but also resulted in him being called a liar by his health care provider (Drake 2016).

Comprehensive sexuality education (#10)

> Older people have the right to education and comprehensive sexuality education. Comprehensive sexuality education must be age appropriate, scientifically accurate, culturally competent and grounded in human rights, gender equality and a positive approach to sexuality, ageing and pleasure.

A confluence of factors put transgender people who transition in mid-life at particular vulnerability for sexually transmitted diseases. The marriages and partnerships of many such individuals break up when one partner transitions (59% of those 65+), potentially putting the transgender elders in a dating pool they may have been out of for decades (National Center for Transgender Equality 2011). They have certainly heard about HIV and sexually transmitted infections, but often what they heard had no relevance to them because the risk was promoted as being mostly to people of a different sexual orientation, race, and/or gender. Very few know that surgically constructed vaginas and vaginas exposed to testosterone may be particularly vulnerable to tears and, therefore, infection. Moreover, some mid-life transitioners are so eager to be sexually affirmed in their "new" gender that they may take unusual risks. One elder told the authors (Cook-Daniels & Munson 2010):

I only negotiate for BDSM play in the beginning to find someone who will allow me to serve and submit myself to them. I negotiate safer sex opposite maybe what I should but actually I want a man to cum in me and not use condoms as I feel a great need and desire for the seed of a man I guess much like a woman desiring to get pregnant. Once I have a partner I do whatever pleases Him.

Clearly, as much as transgender elders need and want comprehensive sexuality education that is transgender-specific, this has not yet been addressed.

Relationships (#11)

Older people have the right to choose whether or not to marry and to enter freely and with full and free consent into marriage, partnership or other similar relationships. All persons are entitled to equal rights entering into, during, or at dissolution of marriage partnership or other similar relationship without discrimination or exclusion of any kind. This right includes equal entitlements to social welfare and other benefits regardless of the form of relationships.

In many countries, transgender elders and their partners do not have the right to marry. Indeed, in some countries, married transgender people are required to divorce their spouses in order to access transition-related medical care (Ghoshal & Knight 2011). Where same-sex marriage is not allowed, couples may be unable to marry even if they appear to be heterosexual, if the one partner's transgender status is known and the official or court involved believes transgender people can only ever be the sex they were assigned at birth.

Particularly abandoned are the partners of transitioning people. There is no handbook on how to save a marriage when one member of the couple undergoes a gender transition. Furthermore, many transgender support organizations exclude non-trans people, including partners. The lack of resources, information, and support is likely responsible for the high rate of marriage break-ups reported by transgender people: 27% in the last available study (James et al. 2016).

Freedom of thought, opinion and expression (#12)

Older people have the right to freedom of thought, opinion and expression regarding sexuality and the right to express their own sexuality through, for example, appearance, communication and behaviour with due respect to the rights of others.

Very few countries currently give transgender people full rights to name themselves, choose their gender expression, and have identification documents in their correct name and gender. In many countries, these rights are limited and/or controlled by gatekeepers such as physicians, psychotherapists, judges, and others. An extreme example is Ukraine, which mandates that transgender individuals undergo in-patient psychiatric assessment up to 45 days in length, coerced sterilization, numerous medical tests, and "a humiliating in-person evaluation by a government commission to further confirm the diagnosis of 'transsexualism' and authorize the change in legal documents" (Ghoshal & Knight 2011).

In other countries, being transgender is explicitly or practically outlawed. "Posing" as the opposite sex is against the law in many countries, while other states persecute transgender people through laws criminalizing "same-sex" conduct (Ghoshal & Knight 2011). Even in countries where transgender people have some measure of acceptance, a lack of non-discrimination laws may effectively undermine freedom of expression. In the U.S., there are few federal protections for transgender people and just a patchwork of state and local laws. As a result of this legal discrimination, the unemployment rate among transgender people is twice as high as among the general public; one-fifth have been denied a home or apartment because they are transgender; and 53% have been disrespected or verbally harassed in a place of public accommodation (James et al. 2015).

Freedom of association and peaceful assembly (#13)

> *Older people have the right to peacefully organize, associate, assemble, demonstrate and advocate including about sexuality, sexual health and sexual rights.*

Because transgender individuals make up such a small percentage of the population (estimates range from .6% to 1%; Flores et al. 2016) and frequently do their best to not be recognized as transgender, organizing and assembling transgender elders is a difficult task. The advent of the internet was a huge breakthrough, as it allowed individuals struggling with gender-related feelings to search for and find information. The internet also helped such individuals find each other, a task that social media made even easier. One of the first (if not the earliest) was ElderTG, a peer support email listserv for transgender people age 50+ that was founded in 1998. It has continuously maintained at least 100 international subscribers and hosted up to two dozen messages per day. There are also now Facebook pages and other social media sites devoted specifically to older transgender people.

It is important to note, however, that given how many basic human rights transgender elders are still trying to achieve and how much violence and discrimination they must counteract, it is likely that sexual health and sexual rights will not be at the top of transgender elders' organizing agenda for some time.

Participation in public and political life (#14)

> *Older people are entitled to an environment that enables active, free and meaningful participation in and contribution to the civil, economic, social, political and other aspects of human life at local, national, regional and international levels. In particular, older people are entitled to participate in the development and implementation of policies that determine their welfare including their sexuality and sexual health and that influence the design of health and aged care services.*

Very few democracies have elected transgender officials. Transgender people who have gained employment in governments or other policy-making bodies have typically kept their gender identity or history a secret, to avoid opening themselves to legal discrimination, harassment, and even violence.

This void is rapidly filling. An increasing number of advocacy groups have turned their attention to the policy needs of not just transgender people in general, but specifically of transgender elders. In 2012, for instance, a coalition of ageing and transgender advocates published "Improving the Lives of Older Transgender Adults: Recommendations for Policy and Practice" (SAGE). In addition to publishing policy agendas, transgender advocates have also been successful in convincing public officials to make positive changes. In 2016, for example, U.S. advocates won access to gender confirmation surgeries under Medicare, the health care program for elders.

Justice, remedies and redress (#15)

> Older people have the right to access justice, remedies, and redress for violations of their sexual rights. This requires effective, adequate, accessible and appropriate educative, legislative, judicial and other measures. Remedies include redress through restitution, compensation, rehabilitation, satisfaction and guarantee of non-repetition.

As this chapter has made clear through many examples, transgender elders face a myriad of barriers to exercising not just their sexual rights, but even their very right to exist. The authors are not aware of any country in the world that provides a full range of protections for transgender people in such basic areas of human rights as the ability to name themselves, freely choose their clothing and appearance, obtain and hold employment, access housing, use public accommodations, etc. Countries that do provide some of these rights typically leave transgender people unprotected in many other arenas, with no or little access to remedies such as "restitution, compensation, rehabilitation, satisfaction and guarantee of non-repetition."

Conclusion

The specific case of transgender elders makes a general point quite clear: it is not possible to effectively give sexual rights to people whose basic human rights are still not protected. Transgender elders are still struggling to achieve legal recognition, protection from violence, basic respect, and even – sometimes – acknowledgment of their very existence. In the absence of this basic foundation of rights, achieving sexual rights such as comprehensive sexuality education or being able to peacefully assemble with like others are effectively unattainable.

References

Balzar, C. (2016, March 30). Trans day of visibility press release. *Transgender Europe*. Retrieved from http://tgeu.org/transgender-day-of-visibility-2016-trans-murder-monitoring-update/

Chapman, M.W. (2016, June 2). John Hopkins psychiatrist: Transgender is a 'mental disorder;' sex change 'biologically impossible'. *CNSnews.com*. Retrieved from www.cnsnews.com/news/article/michael-w-chapman/johns-hopkins-psychiatrist-transgender-mental-disorder-sex-change

Cook-Daniels, L. (2016, March 26). Rights v. safety: Exploiting survivors of child molestation. *Huffington Post*. Retrieved from www.huffingtonpost.com/loree-cookdaniels/rights-v-safety-exploitin_b_9523086.html

Cook-Daniels, L., & Munson, M. (2010). Sexual violence, elder abuse, and sexuality of transgender adults, age 50+: Results of three surveys. *Journal of GLBT Family Studies, 6:2.* 142–177.

Cook-Daniels, L., & Munson, M. (2016). First do no harm: Eight tips for addressing violence against transgender and gender non-binary people. *FORGE*. Retrieved from http://forge-forward.org/wp-content/docs/do-no-harm-8-tips-addressing-violence-FINAL.pdf

Drake, T. (2014). *"I'll be damned if I'm going to be buried a girl." Gender transition gives HIV+ trans man reason to live.* [Video]. Retrieved from https://imfromdriftwood.com/teo_drake/

Feinberg, L. (1996). *Transgender warriors: Making history from Joan of Arc to RuPaul.* Boston, MA: Beacon Press.

Feldman, J. (2014, January 15). Fox's Dr. Keith Ablow: "I am not convinced" being transgender is real. *Mediaite.com*. Retrieved from www.mediaite.com/online/fox%E2%80%99s-dr-keith-ablow-%E2%80%98i-am-not-convinced%E2%80%99-being-transgender-is-real/

Flores, A.R., Herman, J., Gates, G., & Brown, T. (2016). How many adults identify as transgender in the United States? *Williams Institute*. Retrieved from http://williamsinstitute.law.ucla.edu/wp-content/uploads/How-Many-Adults-Identify-as-Transgender-in-the-United-States.pdf

Ghoshal, N., & Knight, K. (2011). Rights in transition: Making legal recognition for transgender people a global priority. *Human Rights Watch*. Retrieved from www.hrw.org/world-report/2016/rights-in-transition

Grant, J.M., Mottet, L., Tanis, J., Harrison, J., Herman, J.L., & Keisling, M. (2011). *Injustice at every turn: A report of the national transgender discrimination survey.* Washington, DC: National Center for Transgender Equality and National Gay and Lesbian Task Force.

Harrison-Quintana, J., & Herman, J.L. (2013). Still serving in silence: Transgender service members and veterans in the National Transgender Discrimination Survey. *LGBTQ Policy Journal*. Retrieved from http://williamsinstitute.law.ucla.edu/wp-content/uploads/Harrison-Quintana-Herman-LGBTQ-Policy-Journal-2013.pdf

James, S.E., Herman, J.L., Rankin, S., Keisling, M., Mottet, L., & Anafi, M. (2016). *The report of the 2015 U.S. transgender survey.* Washington, DC: National Center for Transgender Equality.

McHugh, P. (2016, May 13). Transgender surgery isn't the solution. *The Wall Street Journal*. Retrieved from www.wsj.com/articles/paul-mchugh-transgender-surgery-isnt-the-solution-1402615120

National Center for Transgender Equality (2011). Data set from the National Transgender Discrimination Study, analyzed by age bracket. Provided to the authors.

Psychiatry expert: "Scientifically there is no such thing as transgender." (2013, January 15). *Lifesitenews.com*. Retrieved from www.lifesitenews.com/news/psychiatry-expert-scientifically-there-is-no-such-thing-as-transgender

RAINN (n.d.). *Perpetrators of sexual assault: Statistics (n.d.) RAINN*. Retrieved from www.rainn.org/statistics/perpetrators-sexual-violence

Williams, C. (2014). Fact checking Janice Raymond: The NCHCT report. *BruceDocumentBlog*. Retrieved from http://brucedocumentblog.blogspot.com/2016_06_01_archive.html

7

INTERSEX AGEING AND (SEXUAL) RIGHTS

J.R. Latham and M. Morgan Holmes

Introduction

Most research concerning intersexed people focuses on infants, children and adolescents, on variations visible at birth or on surgical and hormonal interventions that conform intersexed variations to normative expectations of sex and gender. Overwhelmingly, intersex research is clinical and produced by doctors, though there is a growing movement of intersex criticism, much of which challenges the accounts and interventions of clinicians in the lives of intersexed people. Yet, neither the concept of *ageing* intersexed nor the experiences of people fitting that category have, until now, received scholarly attention (Talley & Casper 2012). In large part, we believe this is due to the medical notion that intersex variations are problems of childhood, which can be fixed by hormonal and surgical interventions. Against this view, we argue that intersex is a life-long difference, and medical interventions aimed at normalising intersexed differences can and do harm the people they purport to help. This chapter explores intersexed ageing and sexual rights through the data collected from a small, qualitative study conducted in Australia by one of the authors (JRL), who sought to document the experiences and needs of older intersexed people in partnership with Organisation Intersex International (OII) Australia (see Latham & Barrett 2015a). As there is very little research available that documents intersexed people's own experiences of ageing, these narratives provide an important insight into thinking about the issues and difficulties ageing intersexed people face, while acknowledging the vast range of intersex variations and individual experiences. We also draw on the 2012 documentary film *Intersexion*, which presents the testimonies of more than 20 intersexed people from around the world. Together, these two projects give us a place to start to discuss the sexual rights, needs and experiences of ageing intersexed people. In particular, we consider the ways medical interventions, which are often unnecessary, shape intersexed people's experiences of ageing and sexuality.

We use the term 'intersexed' as shorthand for 'intersexualized', by which we mean to emphasise the process through which some persons are subject to medicalisation and pathologisation that shapes both external and self-perception for those who experience diagnosis and management for an intersex biological trait. The concept of active intersexualization (which turns a neutral difference into a pathology) is fully developed by Lena Eckert (2009). We have chosen to avoid the use of 'disorders of sex development' (DSD) as a term that the American medical community developed in 2006 with minimal input from intersex persons themselves (see Lee et al. 2006). Instead, we retain the use of 'intersex' out of respect for and alliance with the work of international activists and advocates to destigmatise intersex and to reclaim the name as one of pride and self-determination (see Holmes 2009). The research literature from clinical practice on ageing and intersex does, however, use DSD, and this literature is represented in our bibliography.

MMH: As one of the few researchers whose work on intersex straddles the formal world of academic scholarship and the more informal, haphazard world – literally a global effort now – of intersex activism that has been carried out by a small but growing number of people running largely on self-financed, small budgets, I am in the unique position to come to this work on intersexed ageing and sexual rights as one of the culpable parties who was absolutely not thinking, in my mid-twenties, about what our long-term healthcare needs would be. To be fair to the relatively nascent field of critical intersex studies, and the largely unfunded network of activists and support groups around the world, two very real considerations have influenced and extended the absence of research in this area of sexual rights of intersexed persons as we age. In no hierarchised order these two features are: 1) a lack of funding and access to populations for follow-up on long-term needs (a consequence of both medical and academic structures that have formed obstacles to developing research); and, 2) the fact that so many of us have literally moved from young adulthood to middle-age along with the movement, and so the concern for the long-term was not the most pressing one when we first set out. How far we have travelled, both in time and in thinking. When I was first writing about intersex and proposing to take up research in a women's studies PhD, I was denied entry on the grounds that 'intersex was not a women's studies concern'. I went, therefore, into an interdisciplinary PhD that did not define its concerns in such a limited fashion, and have in the 20 years since, seen greater interest, acceptance, and funding arrive from a variety of sources, including those in more broadly conceptualised feminist/ gender studies fields.

Much older now and staring down the surgical green corridor of my own ageing, I aver that sexual rights for intersexed persons are often overlapping with the sexual rights of women as much as they are for those who identify outside of a simple male-female divide, and are also – albeit less frequently – a matter for persons who have been both intersexed by medicine and shoe-horned into a male social role.

JRL: I came to this work out of another project on transgender Australians' experiences of ageing (see Latham & Barrett 2015b). Both were tied together due to the financial restrictions of a limited budget, though I argued for (and achieved) their disentanglement, making this project's budget miniscule. As a transgender man who does intersex research, I fear that I contribute to the confusion and conflation of these two groups. There is a tendency among some trans people to claim to be 'intersex', presumably seeking a biological 'cause' for their transsexuality. While I understand the sentiment, these kinds of identity claims miss the point of what 'being intersexed' means and, often, costs. Yet I firmly believe there are useful ways trans and intersex politics can be, and must be, mobilised in coalition.

Addressing the sexual rights of older intersexed people

The sexual rights of older people as they have been described by Barrett and Hinchliff (Chapter 2, this volume) have some specific implications and considerations for intersexed people. Older intersexed people are living with the consequences of how potentially all such sexual rights have been violated, perhaps especially 'the right to equality and non-discrimination' (1) and 'the right to autonomy and bodily integrity' (3). Indeed, many sexual rights have been denied to them for their entire lives. In this way, thinking about how we can care for older intersexed people requires considering the ongoing implications of these violations, as well as how these rights can be protected in the future. Due to the extraordinary dearth of intersex research, we must propel our attendance to sexual rights through a broader analysis of health-care and medical treatment for intersexed older people.

The interview data

Two intersexed people, aged between 55 and 65, were interviewed about their experiences of ageing ('Robert', who has an XXY chromosomal pattern and 'Klinefelter syndrome', and 'Pat', who has congenital adrenal hyperplasia [CAH] – both pseudonyms). An open-ended interview structure was used to allow participants to speak about their concerns, guided minimally by the interviewer. Both participants spoke at length about their sexual lives and identities, and their histories of medical interventions. Both were subject to medical interventions (surgeries and hormone regimes) as children and young adults that were largely if not exclusively cosmetic (not life-saving). They did not consent to these interventions. Indeed, they felt coerced into them, regretted that they had been subjected to them and experienced ongoing negative impacts on their lives. The interview transcripts were shared with MMH after being de-identified. We each independently coded the transcripts for emerging themes and then discussed our findings.

Although *some* hormone treatments are crucial for saving the lives of *some* inter-sexed persons, others serve the purpose of effecting a cosmetic change (towards stereotypical sex characteristics) and maintenance of that change. A person like Pat requires hormone management for salt-wasting metabolic complications in CAH, but may not be concerned about trying to suppress other effects of high andro-gen levels (such as muscle density, height and hair distribution). Because many intersexed persons are not told the purpose of their medications, they may cease taking them or try taking new ones without information about possible medical complications. Both participants expressed concern about how little was known or understood about their intersex variations, including by health professionals. More than this, both worried about the effects on their health *of the medical interventions* they had endured.

Robert recounted his history of medical interventions that shaped his body and self-image, and lamented being coerced by medical professionals into testosterone therapy to 'make him a man'. Robert is accepting of his intersex status, but has difficulty finding other men to share his life – and be sexual – with. He finds the gay men in his city to be ignorant of intersex differences and unaccepting of the ways his body looks and functions differently from other men. He described sexual encounters in which he was accused of 'being a transsexual', and expressed frus-tration by this conflation of intersex with being trans. Pat described gender as an oppressive force that has only hurt her, and worries about the effects of a lifetime of medical interventions on her ageing body. While she follows emerging research and talks to many people about being intersexed, including health professionals, she cannot find information about healthy ageing that is relevant to her.

Intersex ageing: a new population

To speak of intersex ageing concerns is very much a product of recent developments in medicine. One might sum it up by asserting the paradox that some of us (those born with bodies that do not conform to the contemporary binary biological sex model of male/female) have always grown old, but 'we' (those understood as inter-sex) have not always existed.

While there have always been 'older people', there have not always been older *intersex* people who could have understood themselves as such, because the *bio-logical* (rather than the mythological) categorisation of 'hermaphrodites' arose only fairly recently in European history, and the conceptual category of 'intersex' was not developed until the early 20th century (see Dreger 2000; Holmes 2008; Reis 2012 for this history). Prior to the arrival of statist, interventionist and managerial catego-ries developed in the biopolitic that has increasingly informed our self-governance as particular kinds of subjects, Euro-American records were simply not interested in anatomy in the ways that census, citizenship and migration data came to track subjects from the late 19th century forward. The absence of a historical record for intersex persons has not only to do with the issue of sex taxonomies intersecting with governmentality (see Tremain 2001), but it has also to do with the combination of certain health vulnerabilities that made survival past infancy unlikely for some. Those who died in infancy or childhood may have died from associated metabolic crises that would have been catastrophic before mid-20th-century endocrinology provided both identification and treatment options for metabolic regulation. This was explained by Pat, who reports:

> When I was born, the chemical that they used to manage salt-wasting congenital adrenal hypoplasia really wasn't available in Australia and if my salt-wasting had've been extreme salt-wasting, I would've died. Luckily I don't have chronic salt-wasting. When the chemicals became available to manage salt-wasting I was amongst the first users.

By contrast, those who died at a typical age but who may have been discovered on autopsy to have had internal testes, despite a typical female phenotype, are likely to have lived understanding themselves as fairly ordinary (if incapable of reproduction) women for their entire lives. Finally, the 'iatrogenic hermaphrodites' thought to be the result of various drugs used on pregnant women in the mid-20th century present an historically anomalous population that is only now reaching middle age. Moreover, many of the other intersex diagnostic categories (e.g. XXY, Klinefelter Syndrome, Mayer-Rokitansky-Küster-Hauser Syndrome [MRKH], Partial Androgen Insensitivity Syndrome [PAIS]) might have produced subjects who considered themselves to be somewhat remarkable men or women, but they would not have understood themselves until recently as *intersex*, for the concept simply did not exist.

In addition to the developments of medicine and changing demands of the state to categorise subjects according to sex, or to 'fix' intersex in order to make the exceptional fit the rule, there are other reasons that the ageing intersexed population around the world is a new phenomenon. Across many times and cultures, any infant perceived as sexually ambiguous would be put to death in infancy, or ejected from the mainstream. Indeed, a delegate to the intersex forum at the International Lesbian, Gay, Trans and Intersex Association (ILGA) 2012 conference held in Stockholm reported that in areas of West Africa, infants apprehended at birth by midwives as intersex continue to 'routinely have their necks snapped' by the midwives who then tell the mothers that the babies were stillborn.

These historical points add up to a necessary observation that while we have had a population of lesbian, gay and gender-nonconforming older persons, intelligible as such, since the mid-19th century in Euro-American contexts, the arrival of a population of older intersexed persons presents a new population with unique healthcare needs. Moreover, with the extension of Euro-American medical models into developing regions and former colonies, consideration of the global position of intersex human rights is long overdue. Looking forward is, therefore, not something to be done in isolation or from the perspective of pure conjecture. Even the endocrinologists most likely to be working with patients now acknowledge that 'Few sound evidence-based data are available to guide

HRT administration [. . .] in adulthood in [intersexed] individuals,' and add with some hesitation that 'new formulations may give better perspectives for the future' (Hiort & Ahmed 2014, p. 149).

With technical advances in medicine in the latter half of the 20th century, various intersexualizing diagnoses became more common. Consequently, a population of people are now entering early old age with little to no information about what that means. Many of this population have histories of non-consensual medical interventions and are living with the ongoing effects, physically and emotionally, of those interventions. Additionally, they can struggle to address their ongoing health needs because they have been lied to, or had information withheld, by various clinicians over their life histories as patients.

Understanding intersex needs from a life history perspective

Our analysis is informed by what Elder and colleagues (2003) describe as 'life course' theory, meaning that while the histories of people's lives are important, their ongoing needs are shaped by events that exceed the limits of particular stages such as birth and death. Our data are largely provided through interviews and documents that provide life histories – that is, accounts of events that have already happened. However, our data approach the life-course perspective in that they provide accounts of needs, both current and anticipated, informed in part by previous experience.

For some time there has been a vocal and global movement of intersexed persons who identify their experiences of childhood medicalisation as severely traumatising (see Chase 2006), which we may frame as the violation of many sexual rights. Many report that these traumas impair their ability to develop trusting relationships, including with a primary care physician and, thus, they are not receiving adequate care as they age. Moreover, the trauma is frequently left as an untreated wound because the mental health disciplines have too frequently blamed patients, treating the intersexed as though we have simply 'failed' to assimilate properly to our assigned sexes/genders, and have presented obdurate non-compliance as patients. Mani Bruce Mitchell makes this point in *Intersexion*:

> We were part of a generation of children who have been surgically and hormonally assigned to fit neatly into male or female. A generation who are left traumatized and damaged.
>
> *(Intersexion 2012)*

With the knowledge of the often emotionally traumatising and/or physically damaging histories, advocates have been lobbying for change. The past couple of years have seen significant steps toward the official recognition of the sexual and health rights of intersexed persons. The Council of Europe Commissioner for Human Rights (CECHR) issued a statement with eight fundamental recommendations to act on globally. We are interested in the present needs and rights of intersexed persons who have, inevitably, been approached and treated under protocols now widely understood to have been traumatising and in violation of their rights as children who were denied the ability to exercise their 'developing autonomy' (Benson 2005; Greenberg 2005; Holmes 2005; Redick 2005).

We are therefore interested in particular in three provisions laid out in the CECHR report: First, that sex characteristics be included in sex/gender discrimination and hate crime legislation (provision 5). Second, that there is an urgent need to improve both professional education and public awareness about the issues faced by intersexed people, which includes the active participation of intersexed people in research (provision 7). And third, "The human rights violations intersex people have suffered in the past should be investigated and publicly acknowledged and remedied. Ethical and professional standards, legal safeguards and judicial control should be reinforced to ensure future human rights compliance" (provision 8; Agius 2015, pp. 9–10).

Chronic health considerations

Our interview participants identified a need for services to be tailored to suit the particulars of their own healthcare needs going forward into 'old age'. Informing their observations about tailored services, both Pat and Robert discussed concerns for chronic health considerations they anticipated encountering or were already experiencing. For example, Pat, who has a form of CAH that includes a difficulty metabolising salt and producing cortisol and aldosterone, observed that salt-wasting is a chronic health concern that she has been made personally responsible for managing but may not always be able to manage alone. In addition, Pat reported that because of the ongoing influence of the hormonal dysregulation that is a feature of CAH, she has experienced a somewhat masculinised appearance that can provoke hostility in others. This gives Pat cause for concern when anticipating a future in which more permanent care might be required:

> [A]s an ageing intersex person . . . if I end up in a position where I'm showered by somebody else and my body is in its naked state a visibly different body, I think how's that going to play out around the nursing home . . . and do I, you know, end up spending the last years of my life in a kind of living hell as a queer person – and I've had plenty of it, I can tell you plenty of it over my life, as being exhibit number one.

Robert reported that due to his intersex physiology, he feels vulnerable to a future marked by sub-standard care and hostility:

> With my condition I've never been able to work full-time and so I don't have any savings, so I wouldn't be able to purchase a unit or anything like that, [. . .] I fear I'd end up in one of those kinds of wards where, I might have to share, and that's one of the problems – one of my greatest fears.

Robert's worries about his future care and residential circumstances are rooted in a history similar to Pat's, in which normative demands to appear typically gendered as male (in Robert's case) or as female (in Pat's case) led to traumatic interactions that included a range of negative responses to their perceived 'deviance' from gender norms. These negative responses in clinical and social service settings ranged from threats of violence to hostile accusations and conjectures about their personal lives and denials of service.

Prejudices

Both Robert and Pat described encountering social prejudices within medical contexts and elsewhere, particularly homophobia and transphobia, as well as intersex-specific discrimination. For example, Pat experienced the administrative difficulties and barriers of being construed as within a same-sex couple, as she articulated:

> How can a person whose sex is unknown, who they struggled with so much they had to do surgery and all that sort of stuff to give me any sex at all, how can I be a lesbian? I mean what does same-sex mean for an intersex person? [. . .] I had to fight for three years to have the law changed, so that my partner could get my super[annuation] if I die.

In particular, both interviewees felt harmed by the assumption that intersex is a disorder that can be fixed, rather than a life-long difference. This assumption is *practiced in medicine.* Yet the ageing experiences of intersexed people actively contest the notion that intersex *is* an issue of children and that normalising interventions solve those issues.

The ongoing chronic health issues of intersexed adults, as well as the emotional consequences of previous interventions, counter the assumption that intersex *is* a disorder that can be fixed (in childhood), as well as the treatment trajectory that it condones. Robert stressed the need for medicine to take account of the realities of intersexed lives: 'they're still stuck in binary male, female, heterosexual, homosexual, and they just don't recognise that there are people who exist outside or between those binaries.' Robert described the hormonal therapy he was prescribed as a turning point in his life that he profoundly regrets:

> If I had known about intersex stuff then and my rights, I would never have started the hormone therapy because it just turned me into somebody that I'm not. . . . I regret it because I would have preferred to live as an androgynous person, sure I was impotent, but I'm still not able to enjoy sex.

This kind of regret contributes to suspicion of medical professionals and mistrust of their advice.

Both Pat and Robert address issues of being subject to decades of insensitive treatment for various ongoing health concerns that are features of their intersex differences. Pat has required metabolic support to manage her CAH throughout her life and yet reports that with each change in endocrinologist she would find that she was 'one of the few people like me that the professional has seen, certainly the oldest one . . . and you know, it excites all this curiosity like a side show. And a lifetime of that is very wearing.' Pat feels, and we agree, that clinicians owe something better than treating intersexed people as curiosities or professional opportunities. The autonomy and bodily integrity of intersexed persons needs to be respected no less than anyone else, and as Pat observed, 'by way of apology [for a lifetime of negative encounters] they should try and do stuff that will at least make our old age a bit better than our childhood and our youth.' The 'stuff' to which Pat refers is an obligation to become informed about the subfields in endocrinology and reproductive medicine that would make these encounters more respectful and avoid emotionally invasive interrogations and examinations. Clinicians should thus be prepared and informed, and able to listen to the particulars that intersexed adults need. The implication is that a 'universal approach' will not work for care provision, and that instead the standard of care ought to require that services be tailored to the needs determined by each intersexed person.

Intersex services

Unsurprisingly, one of the points emphasised by both Robert and Pat was the need for intersex-specific medical education, research and services. Robert described being misdiagnosed with an endocrinal deficiency in his young adulthood and 'being pumped full of testosterone [to] only get about 10 per cent of the benefits'. Robert highlighted the importance of being able to identify intersex variations and the fatal risks of medically treating intersex people without proper understanding of their specific needs. 'Before I was diagnosed,' Robert explains, 'I was seen by an endocrinologist who was an idiot and nearly killed me, literally.' The experience of being given testosterone and told to be a 'real man', a social imposition beyond his biological limits, was experienced by Robert as traumatic. In addition, when Robert reported his concern about the regime not working to his doctors, he was told 'it's probably your imagination'. Having his experience belittled on top of what he was already going through caused Robert to have, in his words, 'a nervous breakdown'. Robert described how this kind of ignorance was a constant in his encounters with medical professionals: 'I just feel uncomfortable trying to explain, you try to explain who you are and they look at you as though you're some kind of an idiot or that you're mad or that you're confused.' Although Robert's experiences clearly contravene statements on best practice for patient rights, the combination of paternalism and ignorance he is subjected to points to the urgent need for medical education on intersex variations that, at its core, values respect for self-determination.

Two consequences of thinking that intersex is a medical problem of children, which can be 'fixed' by normalising interventions, are that it erases the experiences of intersexed adults and silences the trauma of enduring those interventions (especially before the age of consent. On the contrary, intersexed adults are often treated as though they should be grateful). Furthermore, this way of thinking *forecloses the need for ongoing services*, specifically services for intersexed *adults as they age*. We surmise this is because it would equate to an admission that intersex interventions at best have not 'worked' and at worst are damaging and traumatising. This problem was identified by Pat, who said: 'They kind of do all this stuff when you're a kid to fix you up and send you on your way as a fixed-up person.' A third effect of treating intersex variations in this way is that intersexed adults are relegated to paediatric services. This was experienced by Pat as humiliating, 'It's wonderful, you know, being sent along to a room, you know, it's a waiting room with mothers and babies [. . .] an appropriate endocrinologist for adult intersex people is really hard to come by.'

Pat in particular found it impossible to discover how her experience of ageing would be affected by her intersex differences. Moreover, she was concerned that the decades of under-researched medical interventions she has been subjected to would continue to cause her harm in her later years, to unknown effects. Pat struggled to find a doctor who could advise her about these issues. As Pat explained: 'I really worry about, you know, should I continue on with the stuff [medication] that they've been giving me all my life, is this good for me, bad for me, do I feel I need it, and they don't know or don't say.' While we recognise the importance of preventing unnecessary cosmetic surgeries on infants and other minors, it is equally important that the lives of those who are living with the ongoing effects of these traumatising interventions be attended to, urgently. This was emphasised by Pat:

> The focus is on children and young people, it's like we never grow up. . . . Nobody sees how we manage as adults, how all those interventions have played out for us over a lifetime. And a lot of those interventions, like with me, I was subjected to some really primitive interventions that were around in the '50s, and their response to how my life has played out, my whole life, is, 'Things are much better now, we don't do that anymore.' But hang on a minute, you did it to me, and this is a real life, this is me, this is a living person, *this is my whole life.*

It is important to note that while it may be the case that certain *surgical* techniques have improved, medical interventions that seek to 'normalise' intersexed bodies risk inflicting the same *emotional* damages. In particular, sexual possibilities (especially of pleasure) are overwhelmingly disregarded in the service of *aesthetic social norms and functions* (i.e. urinating from the 'right place' or (hetero)normative sexual intercourse). The shame that invariably accompanies these kinds of sexual or genital interventions has ongoing consequences throughout the sexual lives of intersexed adults (see Morland 2009). This point is emphasised by Mitchell, who describes, 'For me, I haven't had a loving relationship. After all, I was a child being told my body was so horrendous and so not ok it had to have pieces cut off it' (*Intersexion* 2012).

Many of the people appearing in *Intersexion* describe the shame of hiding their differences and being made to lie about 'vacationing' when they were in hospital for surgeries. These practices make intersexed children vulnerable, taught to lie and to keep secret differences about themselves. This makes intersexed children especially vulnerable to abuse and to remaining silent about that abuse, a fact brought to the fore by Mitchell:

> Our genitals have been touched right from when we are little. We've been taught never to talk about our different bodies and so sexual predators are very good at picking out children that would make good victims.
>
> (*Intersexion* 2012)

Gina Wilson elaborated on Mani's point and explained that her lifetime of abuse 'by more than one person' centred around her difference. Wilson, who was being 'raised as a male' but 'dressed as a female', was abused as a female. The abuse consisted of photographing 'that difference about me' (Intersexion 2012).

Another unexpected consequence of hormonal interventions is discussed by intersex human rights advocate David Cameron Strachan who, like Robert, was forced onto a testosterone regime to 'make him look like a real man', which he hated. 'I wasn't really aware of what it was going to do to me. What it did do to me that I liked was it made me really horny. By 1981 I was infected with HIV because I was having lots of sex with lots of different people. Then in 1998 I was diagnosed with AIDS' (*Intersexion* 2012). Beyond the more obvious physical consequences of surgeries, these are important effects of medical interventions, which need to be recognised and researched in order to inform appropriate and effective healthcare.

Conclusions and recommendations

Our analysis of interviews with Robert and Pat, as well as the documentary *Intersexion*, confirms and expands upon the reports from life histories provided by intersexed persons who contributed to the *Intersex in the Age of Ethics* collection (Dreger 1999). These interviews mark some of the first to specifically address the rights and needs of intersexed adults who are at the start of 'old age' and considering their futures. Our contribution here provides a sense of the long-term costs and persistent problems in treatment approaches that intersexed persons still confront.

The introduction of life-long vulnerabilities that are secondary to prejudice, to harmful interventions that have impaired physical function and/or radically disrupted self-perception have left intersexed people with fears of harassment and the potential for further experiences of violence (whether physical or emotional), and living with material constraints that limit their options as they age. We cannot continue to treat intersex as though it is a problem for paediatric medicine, and one that is resolved – rather than produced and/or exacerbated – in childhood. Ongoing prejudices from care providers, in social service venues and in the institutions that intersexed people rely upon present threats to the health and well-being of a group that is already vulnerable to social isolation and more complex health considerations than most people anticipate as they age.

The combination of current clinical practices of intersex treatment (as a physical problem that can be fixed in childhood) coupled with an almost universal failure to educate health practitioners about intersex variations and a complete lack of healthcare research and long-term studies in experiences of intersexed people leaves us almost overwhelmed by the sheer scope of issues this chapter has introduced that need to be urgently addressed. To begin, we suggest the following interpretation of Barrett and Hinchliff's sexual rights:

TABLE 7.1 The sexual rights of older intersexed people

1. The right to equality and non-discrimination	1. Respect for intersex as a human difference
3. The right to autonomy and bodily integrity	3. Value self-determination above social aesthetic norms of male or female
7. The right to the highest attainable standard of health including sexual health	7. Respectful care for intersexed people as they age (age appropriate, intersex specific adult services with knowledgeable professionals)
8. The right to enjoy the benefits of scientific progress and its application	8. Research into the long-term health concerns and needs of intersexed people
11. The right to enter, form and dissolve marriage and other similar types of relationships	11. Equal marriage rights for all couples (phrased as marriage between "two people")
14. The right to participation in public and political life	14. Intersex people must be at the forefront of legislative and medical change. This requires government funding and support for intersex peer support and community groups.
15. The right to access to justice, remedies and redress	15. Recognition of iatrogenic harms experienced by intersexed people (this should include public apologies and compensation)

Another of the under-explored areas of intersex research is the sexual *pleasures* of being intersex. Somewhat unsurprisingly, people not subjected to medical interventions as minors offer accounts of some of the sexual pleasures of their intersex variations. As Hida Viloria explains, 'The clitoris is the only organ on the human body that's specific purpose is pleasure, and it follows that having a large clitoris is just a very positive thing' (*Intersexion* 2012). What remains remarkable to us is that accounts of intersex sexual pleasures such as those described in *Intersexion* seem to have little impact on how surgical and other interventions continue to be considered and practiced. What would intersex medical practice and healthcare look like if *the sexual right to autonomy and bodily integrity* – that is, *self-determination* – were upheld for intersexed people? We dream of a world where that comes to pass.

References

Agius, S 2015, *Human rights and intersex people*, Council of Europe Commissioner for Human Rights, viewed December 1 2015, https://wcd.coe.int/com.instranet.InstraServlet?

command=com.instranet.CmdBlobGet&InstranetImage=2870032&SecMode=1&DocI
d=2346276&Usage=2

Benson, SR 2005, 'Hacking the Gender Binary Myth: Recognizing Fundamental Rights for the Intersexed', *Cardozo Journal of Law & Gender*, vol. 12, no. 1, pp. 31–63.

Chase, C 2006, 'Hermaphrodites with Attitude: Mapping the Emergence of Intersex Political Activism', in S Stryker & S Whittle (eds.), *The Transgender Studies Reader*, Routledge, New York and London, pp. 300–314.

Dreger, AD 1999, *Intersex in the Age of Ethics*, University Publishing Group, Hagerstown, MD.

Dreger, AD 2000, *Hermaphrodites and the Medical Invention of Sex*, Harvard University Press, Cambridge, MA.

Eckert, L 2009, '"Diagnosticism": Three Cases of Anthropological Research into Intersexuality', in M Holmes (ed.), *Critical Intersex*, Queer Interventions, Ashgate, Aldershot, UK, pp. 41–71.

Elder, GH, Johnson, MK & Crosnoe, R 2003, 'The Emergence and Development of a Life Course', in JT Mortimer & MJ Shanahan (eds.), *Handbook of the Life Course*, Springer, New York, pp. 3–19.

Greenberg, JA 2005, 'Intersex and Intrasex Debates: Building Alliances to Challenge Sex Discrimination', *Cardozo Journal of Law & Gender*, vol. 12, no. 1, pp. 99–116.

Hiort, O & Ahmed, SF (eds.) 2014, *Understanding Differences and Disorders of Sex Development (DSD)*, Karger, Basel, Switzerland.

Holmes, M 2005, 'Distracted Attentions: Intersexuality and Human Rights Protections', *Cardozo Journal of Law & Gender*, vol. 12, pp. 127–133.

Holmes, M 2008, *Intersex: A Perilous Difference*, Susquehanna University Press, Selinsgrove PA.

Holmes, M 2009, 'Introduction: Straddling the Past, Present and Future', in M Holmes (ed.), *Critical Intersex*, Queer Interventions, Ashgate, Aldershot, UK, pp. 1–12.

Intersexion 2012, documentary, Ponsonby Productions, Ponsonby, NZ. Produced by John Keir; directed by Grant Lahood.

Latham, JR & Barrett, C 2015a, *'As we age': An Evidence-based Guide to Intersex Inclusive Aged Care Services*, La Trobe University, viewed March 28, 2016.

Latham, JR & Barrett, C 2015b, *'We're people first': Trans Health and Ageing: An Evidence-based Guide to Inclusive Services*, La Trobe University, viewed March 28, 2016.

Lee, P, Houk, C, Ahmed, F & Hughes, L 2006, 'Consensus Statement on Management of Intersex Disorders', *Pediatrics*, vol. 118, no. 2, pp. 488–500.

Morland, I 2009, 'What Can Queer Theory Do for Intersex?', *GLQ: A Journal of Lesbian and Gay Studies*, vol. 15, no. 2, pp. 285–312.

Redick, A 2005, 'What Happened at Hopkins: The Creation of the Intersex Management Protocols', *Cardozo Journal of Law & Gender*, vol. 12, no. 1, pp. 289–296.

Reis, E 2012, *Bodies in Doubt: An American History of Intersex*, Johns Hopkins University Press, Baltimore, MD.

Talley, HL & Casper, MJ 2012, 'Intersex and Aging: A (Cautionary) Research Agenda', in TM Witten & AE Eyler (eds.), *Gay, Lesbian, Bisexual & Transgender Aging: Challenges in Research, Practice & Policy*, Johns Hopkins University Press, Baltimore, MD, pp. 270–289.

Tremain, S 2001, 'On the Government of Disability', *Social Theory & Practice*, vol. 27, no. 4, pp. 617–636.

8

SEXUAL ASSAULT OF OLDER WOMEN

Breaking the silence

Bianca Fileborn, Catherine Barrett, and Karen A. Roberto

Introduction

Despite receiving increasing attention over the past decade, the sexual assault of older women remains a largely hidden and under-recognised phenomenon. With the rising focus on the sexuality and sexual rights of older adults, it becomes ever more pressing to ensure that sexual relations in later life are ethical and mutually consented to. Simultaneously, there has been an emerging public discussion on violence against women, with more public recognition, debate and policy response on this issue than has arguably ever been witnessed. Older women, however, remain largely absent from such discussions, often positioned as 'asexual' (as the Introductory chapter and Chapter 2 illustrated in some detail) and, therefore, unlikely victims of sexual assault. Where the sexual assault of older women is acknowledged, it is typically framed as a form of 'elder abuse', a conceptual category that obscures the gendered power relations that continue to underlie this violence. In the instances where older women are included in research on sexual and intimate partner violence, they tend to be 'lumped' into the amorphous category of the 50+ or 60+ age group. This collapses the diversity of older women and obfuscates the unique or particular experiences of women in different stages of 'old' age. Likewise, the particular role that age plays in mediating experiences of sexual assault tends to be absent as a category of analysis in the sexual assault literature.

For the purposes of this chapter, we take the term 'sexual assault' to mean any behavior of a sexual nature that was not, or could not be, consented to by the victim/survivor. We are concerned with privileging older women's lived experiences of sexual assault and not with any particular legal definition or conceptualisation of this harm. Clearly, the sexual assault of older women directly negates their sexual (and other) rights: with the right to live free from sexual violence or coercion an explicit sexual right. Most notably, sexual assault can remove women's right to autonomy and bodily integrity. It can also deny women the ability to make decisions regarding their sexual relationships and practices. Sexual assault by definition impairs older women's ability to enter into sexual relationships freely and with full consent. It is associated with a range of negative health and psychological outcomes (Cook et al. 2013; Speck et al. 2013). These outcomes may be exacerbated for older victim/survivors (Burgess, Dowdell & Prentky 2000; Burgess & Morgenbesser 2005; Groth 1978), thus preventing older women from achieving the highest attainable level of health and well-being. We take up some of these issues throughout this chapter. In short, sexual assault directly contravenes the sexual rights of older women and must be addressed so that older women can operate as fully actualised sexual citizens.

In this chapter we consider how the sexual assault of older women can be addressed and prevented through the lens of sexual rights. In order to do so, it is important to consider the unique experiences of older women and the ways in which these experiences are shaped by the intersections of gender and age. Viewing sexual assault as an outcome of gendered-power relations and inequality, it must also be situated within 'the system of inequality, based on age, which privileges the not-old at the expense of the old' – though age also intersects and interacts with other power relations (Calasanti, Slevin & King 2006, p. 13). Indeed, according to this theoretical approach, Jones and Powell (2006) argued that we must view older women as being particularly vulnerable to sexual violence, as they are doubly oppressed on account of both their gender and their age. The older body has specific, corporeal realities that shape the ways in which older women experience and are impacted by sexual assault. It is not necessarily helpful to view their experiences as being the same as their younger counterparts (Calasanti, Slevin & King 2006), although they may overlap.

To begin with, we establish what is currently known about the prevalence and incidence of sexual assault against older women. We then move on to consider the ways in which older women's experiences, and responses to those experiences, are shaped by ageism and gender, and establish some of the unique factors that influence the sexual assault of older women. This has particular implications for policy and practice responses to the sexual assault of older women, and we explore some of these in the closing section. While we attempt to touch on issues pertaining to cultural diversity, the bulk of the research conducted to date focuses on the experiences of older women in Western countries. As such, our discussion inevitably centers predominantly on Western women. Additionally, as most research to date has focused on the experiences of heterosexual women – or the sexual orientation of participants is not stated – we focus predominantly on heterosexual women in this chapter. However, we acknowledge that older women in same-sex relationships also experience sexual violence and may have different needs.

What do we know about sexual assault against older women?

In the section that follows we provide an overview of what is currently known about the sexual assault of older women. The bulk of the research conducted to date is concerned with older women in residential aged care settings. It is also clear that older women may have unique needs and experiences depending upon whether they are living in the community or in an aged care setting – though there is also overlap in the experiences of these two groups, and older women can move in and out of community and residential aged care settings (e.g., respite care). As such, we have addressed these two groups of women separately in the ensuing discussion. The research that we discuss here almost certainly underestimates the true prevalence of sexual violence against older women, as others have noted (Ball & Fowler 2008; Cook et al. 2011; Groth 1978; Lea, Hunt & Shaw 2011). Although we elaborate on some of the more specific reasons for this as follows, these studies also suffer from some of the 'global' limitations of sexual assault research, namely that victim/survivors often do not recognise or label their experiences as sexual violence (and thus do not disclose them). Definitions of sexual assault, the research methods used and demographic characteristics of the samples vary across the studies, and thus the scope of experiences identified range greatly between studies.

Women in the community

Prevalence

Older women appear to account for only a small minority of community-dwelling sexual assault victims. For example, police statistics in the United Kingdom indicate that women aged 60 and older constitute 1.7% of all reported sexual offences (Ball & Fowler 2008). According to data from the U.S. Department of Justice (Planty et al. 2013), rates of sexual assault decline with age, with women aged 65 and older experiencing rape and sexual assault at a rate of 0.2 experiences of victimisation per 1,000 members of the population between 2005–2010. In contrast, women aged 12–34 were approximately four times more likely to experience rape or sexual assault.

Self-report studies indicate a similarly low prevalence of sexual assault, with 0.6% of a sample (n = 5777) of community-dwelling older adults in the U.S. reporting having experienced sexual abuse in the past 12 months (Acierno et al. 2010; see also Cannell et al. 2014). Research across Australia and Europe has documented similarly low self-report rates (ABS 2014; Soares et al. 2010). However, older women from socially and economically marginalised groups have been consistently identified as facing a higher risk of experiencing sexual abuse (Amstadter et al. 2011; DeLiema et al. 2012; Melchiorre et al. 2013). This suggests that culturally and economically marginalised women may face a higher risk of sexual assault than their mainstream counterparts do. Research on elder abuse more generally suggests that those from lower socio-economic backgrounds and marginalised communities have lower awareness of what constitutes abuse (Naughton, Drennan & Lafferty 2014). This lack of awareness, lack of social support and lack of financial means may dovetail to create a context of enhanced vulnerability, and reduced likelihood of disclosure.

However, there are also some significant limitations associated with this research. Older women are often excluded from larger prevalence surveys, as in the Crime

Survey for England and Wales with an upper-age limit of 59 (Office for National Statistics 2015), or are combined into a single category of age. For instance, both the Australian Personal Safety Survey (ABS 2006, 2014) and the U.S. Bureau of Statistics (Planty et al. 2013) figures on sexual assault place all women aged 55+ and 65+ respectively into the same category of analysis. These figures are therefore likely to underestimate the true extent of sexual assault against older women and collapse any difference in experience for women in early versus 'deep' old age. Women with cognitive impairment are often excluded from community samples, despite being particularly vulnerable to sexual assault. The barriers that older women face to recognising and reporting their experiences further exacerbate this issue.

Perpetrators

A range of different individuals perpetrate sexual violence against community-dwelling older women across different contexts. Research illustrates that older women are perpetrated against in the context of intimate partner violence – and this violence may begin in later life or be a continuation of an ongoing pattern of violence. Sons and other male family members have also been identified as perpetrators of sexual assault against older women, as have those with caring responsibilities (e.g., health care workers, family members and partners who fulfill the caring role) (Mann et al. 2014). Other studies have documented strangers as a key group of perpetrators (e.g., Cartwright & Moore 1989; Lea, Hunt & Shaw 2011), but research on sexual violence more generally would tend to suggest that this type of victim/offender relationship is rare, with perpetrators much more likely to be known individuals.

Reporting and responses

We know relatively little about the extent to which older women in the community recognise and report their experiences, though it is likely that they face significant barriers to doing so. Sexual assault is widely under-reported across the general population of victim/survivors, with the majority never reporting their experience (ABS 1996; Lievore 2003). For example, in the aforementioned study by Acierno and colleagues (2010), only 16% of individuals who had experienced sexual abuse in the past 12 months reported their experiences to the police. Like most victim/survivors of sexual assault, older women face a range of barriers to identifying and· reporting experiences of sexual violence, including embarrassment, self-blame, fear of the justice system, or feeling that they will not be believed (Lievore 2003, 2005), in addition to barriers related to their age and health status (Fileborn 2016). Such barriers serve as a direct impediment to older women's right to justice and redress for sexual harm.

Older women who have been sexually assaulted by a family member note several reasons for not reporting the assault, including fear that their perpetrator will harm them further; concerns about being placed in a residential aged care facility; concern the family member will go to jail; not believing that help is available; acceptance of a long-standing abusive situation as one that must be tolerated; and not recognising their situation as an abusive one (Roberto 2016). There is very little research on the ways in which others respond to older women when they report or disclose their experiences. Given that dominant discourses construct older women as 'asexual', and sexual assault is often misconstrued as being about sexual desire – older women tend not to be viewed as sexually desirable – it is possible that older women are less likely to be believed when they do report or disclose their experiences. However, we currently lack empirical data to evidence this claim either way.

Residential and aged care settings

Prevalence

Existing research suggests that the prevalence of sexual violence against older women in residential aged care settings (e.g., nursing homes and hostels) is low, similar to their community-dwelling counterparts. For example, Roberto and Teaster (2005) found that incidents of elder sexual abuse make up less than 1% of cases substantiated by the Adult Protective Services (APS) in Virginia (USA). In Australia, where compulsory reporting is in place for residential aged care, the Department of Health (2015) received 426 reports of alleged sexual assault in the 2014–2015 period, although these data exclude perpetrators with cognitive impairments.

Research by Baker, Sugar and Eckert (2009) illustrates that location matters in shaping the experiences of older women who have been sexually assaulted. For women in residential aged care settings, their perpetrators are more likely to abuse their control and authority over the victim rather than to use physical force or coercion, although this is more so the case when the perpetrator is a member of staff. Teaster and Roberto (2003) report that sexually victimised women aged 80 and older were more likely to have experienced multiple types of sexual abuse, suggesting that those in advanced old age may be increasingly vulnerable to sexual victimisation.

There are again limitations associated with this body of research and concerns regarding the extent to which it underestimates the prevalence of sexual assault in these settings. For instance, research in residential aged care tends to be based on reports of sexual assault within a small number of facilities, rather than a broader sample. Currently, there are no available data on the national prevalence of sexual assault in aged care facilities. Again, women in these settings also face significant barriers to recognising and disclosing their experiences (and we expand on this in the next section), suggesting that the sexual assault perpetrated against them often goes unrecognised. Many of these studies rely on the reports and interpretations of staff, meaning that only assaults that are observed are likely to be counted and that sexual assaults by staff are less likely to be reported.

Perpetrators

While a range of individuals may perpetrate against older women in residential aged care settings (including family members, partners and visitors), the two most common categories of perpetrators are members of staff and other residents. There is some debate in the current literature regarding which of these two categories of perpetrator is most common. Some, such as Teaster and Roberto (2003) and Ramsey-Klawsnik et al. (2008), suggest that other residents are the most likely class of perpetrators. Others, such as Payne (2010), have identified staff as the most common group of perpetrators against women in residential aged care settings – and Payne argues that perpetrators may in fact seek employment in these settings in order to gain access to vulnerable women. Certainly, staff wield a significant amount of power and control over residents, and this would enable them to perpetrate with relative impunity in many circumstances. In contrast, other residents may be less able to conceal their behavior from staff and other residents.

Reporting and responses

As indicated previously, women in residential aged care settings can face significant barriers to recognising and reporting any experience of sexual assault. Many older women experience cognitive impairment, disability or other infirmities that can prevent them from being able to directly and coherently communicate their experience to others. However, this does not necessarily mean that these women do not or cannot communicate their experiences, but rather that the ways in which they communicate are ignored or positioned as lacking credibility.

Residents in institutional settings are placed in a relatively powerless position and are often denied control and autonomy over their daily lives and routines (Clark & Fileborn 2011). As a result, residents may have less control over whether or not an assault is reported, particularly if they are dependent upon care staff to make a report on their behalf. Conversely, a lack of control may mean that an assault is reported when the victim/survivor does not want it to be (for example, given the often traumatic nature of the justice system, victim/survivors prefer not to report their experience). There is a considerable power imbalance between people living in residential aged care and members of staff. Given that service providers who perpetrate sexual assault are likely to target older women with dementia or other cognitive impairments, these women are less likely to be believed or viewed as credible. As a result, the staff members may be more able to hide, deny or otherwise cover up their actions. It can also be challenging to establish the absence of consent where sexual activity takes place between residents (Clark & Fileborn 2011; Connolly et al. 2012; Tarzia, Fetherstonghaugh & Bauer 2012), or that the actions of the perpetrator were intentional. Such incidents would often fall outside the remit of the criminal law, although this does not mean that these incidents are unproblematic or that they do not cause harm or distress.

There is evidence to suggest that residential aged care facilities prefer to handle incidents of sexual assault 'in-house' in order to avoid negative attention (Mann et al. 2014; Ramsey-Klawsnik & Teaster 2012; Roberto & Teaster 2005). Facility staff and management can be defensive in the face of sexual assault allegations against staff members or accusations of improper management of allegations (Mann et al. 2014). Residential aged care providers do not always have formal policies or frameworks in place for responding to allegations of sexual assault (Clark & Fileborn 2011; Mann et al. 2014), and this can impede the implementation of an appropriate response to any allegations. Staff may also fear negative ramifications for speaking out about incidents of sexual assault, and this is also likely to act as a barrier to addressing sexual violence within care facilities.

Ageism, gender and sexual assault: considering the unique needs and experiences of older women

The sexual assault of older women is in direct contravention of their sexual rights and must be addressed whenever and wherever it occurs. Older women's experiences of sexual violence are also shaped by both gendered and ageist discourses. In this section, we consider the ways in which such discourses shape women's experiences, and in particular how they contribute towards the occlusion of sexual assault against older women and deny older women their right to access justice or legal remedies.

Health and cognition

Later life can be accompanied by cognitive decline and ailing health, and these factors can increase older women's vulnerability to sexual assault, as well as reducing their perceived 'credibility' in the eyes of bystanders and the justice system. This is not to suggest that older women are inherently vulnerable to sexual assault. Rather, our cultural and social beliefs and attitudes towards ageing actively produce older women as vulnerable, and can enable perpetrators to target and offend against this group with relative impunity (Clark & Fileborn 2011; Mann et al. 2014). Older individuals are often positioned as vulnerable as a result of the assumption that ageing results in cognitive impairment, as much as any actual impairment.

Ironically, the factors that create vulnerability can also negatively impact responses to elder sexual assault from the justice system and others (Poulos & Sheridan 2008). For example, older victims may be easily confused and less able to articulate their experience in a consistent or coherent manner (Burgess, Dowdell & Prentky 2000; Groth 1978; Ramsey-Klawsnik 1991; Speck et al. 2013). As noted earlier, the cognitive and physical impairments that often accompany older age can leave older women more vulnerable to sexual assault on the basis that they are less likely to be believed or less able to communicate and disclose their experience in a coherent way (Burgess & Morgenbesser 2005; Eckert & Sugar 2008; Jones & Powell 2006;

Mann et al. 2014; Payne 2010; Ramsey-Klawsnik 1991; Ramsey-Klawsnik et al. 2008; Ramsey-Klawsnik & Teaster 2012).

When police do interview older victims or undertake some investigation, there are differential outcomes for victims based on their cognitive health. Burgess and Phillips (2006), for example, found that older individuals without dementia who were interviewed by police had more favourable criminal justice outcomes and were more likely to see their cases progressed after an initial complaint had been made. Likewise, Teaster et al.'s (2015) research found that older women without dementia were more likely than their counterparts with dementia to have their cases substantiated. As mentioned previously, for older women in residential aged care settings, sexual assault complaints may be handled 'in-house' rather than in conjunction with law enforcement (Mann et al. 2014; Ramsey-Klawsnik & Teaster 2012; Roberto & Teaster 2005). Older women victim/survivors appear to have differential access to the justice system based upon their cognitive ability and health status and, undoubtedly, a range of other factors such as socio-economic status.

Reported cases of elder sexual abuse analysed by Burgess and Phillips (2006) bring the effect of ageist discourses into sharp relief. One-third of older victims were able to report the sexual abuse they experienced. In the majority of instances, family members, friends or health professionals reported on the victim's behalf. The ability to self-report was significantly limited by having dementia. In short, older individuals with dementia were much less likely to verbally self-report in comparison to older people without dementia. However, older people with dementia in fact *did* disclose through the use of behavioural cues (e.g., being fearful of the perpetrator, showing signs of distress during personal care – see also Burgess & Clements 2006; Burgess, Dowdell & Prentky 2000; Ramsey-Klawsnik 1991; Speck et al. 2013). The issue here seems to be not that women with cognitive impairment are not credible witnesses or are unable to disclose, but rather that the ways in which they do disclose are not heard or recognised. There is a need to develop a more thorough understanding of the ways in which older women with dementia communicate and disclose sexual assault to promote access to justice for these victims (see, for example, Speck et al. 2013). There is also a need to recognise that older women with cognitive impairment can be specifically targeted by perpetrators who are aware of the barriers cognition plays in reporting.

Another significant issue is the extent to which older women may be reliant on their perpetrator to provide them with care, although this issue can also be faced by younger women, particularly those living with a disability (Burgess & Clements 2006; Burgess, Dowdell & Prentky 2000; Clark & Fileborn 2011; Ramsey-Klawsnik 1991; Roberto & Teaster 2005). However, for some women as they age, it becomes more likely that they will need to rely on others to fulfil their care needs (Roberto & Teaster 2005). This dependency can play a role in sexual violence in a number of ways. It may act as a barrier to disclosure, particularly if the older woman is unable to have her care needs met through other individuals or services (Clark & Fileborn 2011; Mann et al. 2014). Being reliant on care services can mean that, in the words of one of Mann et al.'s participants, older women do not 'always have [a] way of picking and choosing who is in their life' (2014, p. 22; see also Burgess & Phillips 2006; Holt 1993). This vulnerability can be further compounded by social and geographical isolation and limited financial means (Burgess & Morgenbesser 2005; Mann et al. 2014). Jones and Powell observe that perpetrators will often 'accompany the elderly victim to healthcare appointments, making it impossible to speak out' (2006, p. 215). Thus, the victim's dependency on the perpetrator further enhances the power and control that the perpetrator is able to enact over their lives.

Conversely, older women may themselves provide care for their perpetrators. Mann et al. (2014), for example, documented older women experiencing unwanted sexual advances from their partners who had dementia. These men were often unaware that they were making repeated demands of penetrative vaginal sex, continued to be prescribed erection-enhancing medications by their doctor, and had little appreciation of the impact their behaviour had on their partner. Experiencing these repeated demands was often highly distressing for the women involved. While we do not suggest that these men were acting with intent, their actions were sexually harmful and impaired older women's sexual rights nonetheless.

Ageism and asexuality

The ageist view of older people as less valuable or worthy can directly impact on how instances of sexual assault of older women are responded to or perceived by others. Mann and colleagues (2014, p. 15) contend that ageist attitudes give rise to the mistaken perception that 'if sexual assaults occur at all . . . it is likely that older women are relatively 'unharmed' by them' – although the basis of such a belief is unclear (see also Holt 1993). Dominant ageist discourses can work to position older women as asexual, rendering the notion that older women could be the victims of sexual violence unimaginable or impossible. It is not our intention here to conflate the issues of sexuality and (perceived) sexual desirability with sexual assault, although these concepts are undoubtedly interrelated. Indeed, as Connolly et al. (2012, p. 45) noted, it is the belief both 'that older people are asexual and that sexual assault constitutes sexual activity' that facilitates and obscures the sexual assault of older women. This perception is further amplified by rape myths depicting victims as young, sexually attractive women – a myth that can mean that older victim/survivors are even less likely to be believed (Cartwright & Moore 1989; Lea, Hunt & Shaw 2011; Vierthaler 2008).

It is currently unclear how ageist discourses pertaining to sexuality and sexist discourses pertaining to ageing might shape how older women understand their own experiences of sexual violence, or the perceptions of family members, health care professionals and so forth. Certainly, the myth that old age is a 'protective' factor against sexual assault is likely to leave many service providers, families and older women themselves unprepared to deal with or identify sexual assault when it occurs.

Cohort sexual culture

The particular cultural context in which current generations of older women grew up is also likely to shape their experiences of, attitudes towards and beliefs about sexual assault. For instance, many older women grew up in a time where sexual violence (or, indeed, sex in general) was not openly discussed or acknowledged (Duncan 2007–2008; Mann et al. 2014; Poulos & Sheridan 2008; Vierthaler 2008), and where legal definitions of sexual violence were limited in comparison to current approaches. For example, many older women will have grown up in a context where rape in marriage was not legally recognised, and sex in marriage was constructed as a woman's 'duty' (Mann et al. 2014; Ramsey-Klawsnik 1991). Marital immunity to rape still exists across many countries and cultural contexts, with UN Women reporting in 2011 that only 52 states explicitly legislate against marital rape. This cultural and legal construct of heterosexual relations continues to position women as vulnerable to sexual violence whilst denying them avenues of legal or other redress.

This raises questions regarding the extent to which older women are likely to recognise or label certain experiences as being sexual violence, or whether they feel able to disclose. For many, sex was a private, taboo topic, and such attitudes may create significant barriers to older women disclosing or identifying their experiences of sexual assault. However, the extent to which older women recognise what constitutes sexual violence remains considerably underexplored and a notable gap in the literature.

Implications for policy, practice and research

How can we move forward from here to ensure that older women's right to be free from sexual violence and coercion is actualised? And how do we ensure women's right to access justice? It is clear from our discussion of the research that significant gaps exist in current knowledge. For example, while it is highly likely that ageist stereotypes regarding older women as 'asexual', or suggesting that the sexual assault of older women is relatively 'harmless', impede the recognition and appropriate responses to the sexual assault of older women, this is yet to be documented through rigorous research efforts. Likewise, we know relatively little of older women's experiences of reporting to the justice system or of their particular support needs. It is difficult to adequately respond to and support older women who have been sexually assaulted when the nature of their experiences has not been fully elucidated.

It is vital to challenge the structural issues of ageism and sexism in preventing the sexual assault of older women. As we have illustrated throughout this chapter, these factors directly enable and excuse the actions of perpetrators by constructing older women as vulnerable and as inherently unreliable narrators of their own lives. In order for the sexual assault of older women to be prevented, or, at the very least, appropriately responded to when it occurs, it is essential that policy and prevention campaigns be inclusive of older women. Older women's experiences must be made visible within our policy and prevention frameworks. Acknowledging older women as the potential victims of sexual assault also demands that residential aged care facilities enact policy and training around this issue. Given that care facilities are steeped in power and control, taking steps to enhance patients' autonomy may assist in preventing sexual assault (Clark & Fileborn 2011).

Community-based responses are also essential here. Although sexual assault is perpetrated by and against individuals, it is taking place within a community context. As such, responses and solutions must include not only older women but also the broader community environment (Roberto et al. 2013). Likewise, it is important to consider how the community can work to break the cycle of silence that so often prevents older women from disclosing or reporting their experiences of sexual assault. It is vital that service providers and the justice system take steps to reach out to older women to communicate that their services are open to, and inclusive of, this segment of the community. This may require the introduction of innovative and flexible practices. For example, being willing to provide services in the homes or residential aged care setting in which older women with limited mobility live. Developing protocols for interviewing older women with cognitive impairment within the justice system would also assist in reducing the likelihood of their experiences being dismissed. Given the wide range of services and service providers who may come into the lives of older women, strategies for preventing and responding to the sexual assault of older women must take a multi-agency, collaborative approach. All services that work with older women need to develop training, policy and screening/intervention protocols to identify and respond to women who are experiencing, or are at risk of experiencing, sexual assault.

Conclusion

The sexual assault of older women constitutes a serious breach of their sexual rights. In order for these rights to be fully realised, we must take the sexual assault of older women seriously and take comprehensive steps to respond to and prevent this violence. Although considerable gains have been made in knowledge and awareness of this issue over the past decade, there is still some way to go in developing the insight required to enable significant change to occur. In the words of Mears (2003, p. 1488), 'violence against older women can no longer be left in the too hard basket'. It is time to take immediate action.

References

Acierno, R, Hernandez, MA, Amstadter, AB, Resnick, HS, Steve, K, Muzzy, W, & Kilpatrick, DG 2010, 'Prevalence and correlates of emotional, physical, sexual, and financial abuse and potential neglect in the United States: The national elder mistreatment study', *American Journal of Public Health*, vol. 100, pp. 292–297.

Amstadter, A, Zajac, K, Strachan, M, Hernandez, M, Kilpatrick, D, & Acierno, R 2011, 'Prevalence and correlates of elder mistreatment in South Carolina: The South Carolina elder mistreatment study', *Journal of Interpersonal Violence*, vol. 26, no. 15, pp. 2947–2972.

Australian Bureau of Statistics 1996, *Women's Safety Survey*, Australian Bureau of Statistics, Canberra.

Australian Bureau of Statistics 2006, *Personal Safety Survey*, Australian Bureau of Statistics, Canberra.

Australian Bureau of Statistics 2014, *Personal Safety Survey*, Australian Bureau of Statistics, Canberra.

Baker, MW, Sugar, NF, & Eckert, LO 2009, 'Sexual assault of older women: Risk and vulnerability by living arrangement', *Sexuality Research & Social Policy*, vol. 6, pp. 79–87.

Ball, HN, & Fowler, D 2008, 'Sexual offending against older female victims: An empirical study of the prevalence and characteristics of recorded offences in a semi-rural English county', *The Journal of Forensic Psychiatry & Psychology*, vol. 19, pp. 14–32.

Burgess, AW, & Clements, PT 2006, 'Information processing of sexual abuse in elders', *Journal of Forensic Nursing*, vol. 2, pp. 113–120.

Burgess, AW, Dowdell, EB, & Prentky, RA 2000, 'Sexual abuse of nursing home residents', *Journal of Psychosocial Nursing & Mental Health Services*, vol. 38, pp. 10–18.

Burgess, AW, & Morgenbesser, LI 2005, 'Sexual violence and seniors', *Brief Treatment & Crisis Intervention*, vol. 5, pp. 193–202.

Burgess, AW, & Phillips, SL 2006, 'Sexual abuse, trauma and dementia in the elderly: A retrospective study of 284 cases', *Victims and Offenders*, vol. 1, pp. 193–204.

Calasanti, T, Slevin, KF, & King, N 2006, 'Ageism and feminism: From "et cetera" to center', *NWSA Journal*, vol. 18, pp. 13–30.

Cannell, MB, Manini, T, Spence-Almaguer, E, Maldonado-Molina, M, & Andresen, EM 2014, 'US population estimates and correlates of sexual abuse of community-dwelling older adults', *Journal of elder abuse & neglect*, vol. 26, no. 4, pp. 398–413.

Cartwright, PS, & Moore, RA 1989, 'The elderly victim of rape', *Southern Medical Journal*, vol. 82, no. 8, pp. 988–989.

Clark, H, & Fileborn, B 2011, 'Responding to women's experiences of sexual assault in institutional and care settings', *ACSSA Wrap*, no. 10, Australian Institute of Family Studies, Melbourne.

Connolly, MT, Breckman, R, Callahan, J, Lachs, M, Ramsey-Klawsnik, H, & Solomon, J 2012, 'The sexual revolution's last frontier: How silence about sex undermines health, well-being, and safety in old age', *Generations*, vol. 36, pp. 43–52.

Cook, JM, Dinnen, S, & O'Donnell, C 2011, 'Older women survivors of physical and sexual violence: a systematic review of the quantitative literature', *Journal of Women's Health*, vol. 20, no. 7, pp. 1075–1081.

Cook, JM, Pilver, C, Dinnen, S, Schnurr, PP, & Hoff, R 2013, 'Prevalence of physical and sexual assault and mental health disorders in older women: Findings from a nationally representative sample', *American Journal of Geriatric Psychiatry*, vol. 21, pp. 877–886.

DeLiema, M, Gassoumis, ZD, Homeier, DC, & Wilber, KH 2012, 'Determining prevalence and correlates of elder abuse using promotores: Low-income immigrant latinos report high rates of abuse and neglect', *Journal of the American Geriatrics Society*, vol. 60, no. 7, pp. 1333–1339.

Department of Health 2015, *2014–15 Report on the operation of the Aged Care Act 1997*, Department of Health, Canberra.

Duncan, J 2007–2008, 'Elder abuse and family violence: Snapshots of violence against women', *Women against Violence*, vol. 20, pp. 18–22.

Eckert, LO, & Sugar, NF 2008, 'Older victims of sexual assault: an underrecognized population', *American Journal of Obstetrics & Gynecology*, vol. 198, pp. 688e1–688e7.

Fileborn, B 2016, 'Sexual assault and justice for older women: A critical review of the literature', *Trauma, Violence & Abuse*, e-pub ahead of print.

Groth, N 1978, 'The older rape victim and her assailant', *Journal of Geriatric Psychiatry*, vol. 11, no. 2, pp. 203–215.

Holt, MG 1993, 'Elder sexual abuse in Britain', *Journal of Elder Abuse & Neglect*, vol. 6, pp. 63–71.

Jones, H, & Powell, JL 2006, 'Old age, vulnerability and sexual violence: Implications for knowledge and practice', *International Nursing Review*, vol. 53, pp. 211–216.

Lea, SJ, Hunt, L, & Shaw, S 2011, 'Sexual assault of older women by strangers', *Journal of Interpersonal Violence*, vol. 26, pp. 2303–2320.

Lievore, D 2003, *Non-reporting and hidden recording of sexual assault: An international literature review*, Australian Institute of Criminology for the Australian Government's Office for Women, Canberra.

Lievore, D 2005, *No longer silent: A study of women's help-seeking decisions and service responses to sexual assault*, Australian Institute of Criminology, Canberra.

Mann, R, Horsley, P, Barrett, C, & Tinney, J 2014, *Norma's project: A research study into the sexual assault of older women in Australia*, Australian Research Centre in Sex, Health and Society, Melbourne.

Mears, J 2003, 'Survival is not enough: Violence against older women in Australia', *Violence against Women*, vol. 9, no. 12, pp. 1478–1489.

Melchiorre, MG, Chiatta, C, Lamura, G, Torres-Gonzales, F, Stankunas, M, Lindert, J, Ioannidi-Kapolou, E, Barros, H, Macassa, G, & Soares, JFJ 2013, 'Social support, socio-economic status, health and abuse among older people in seven European countries', *PLoS One*, vol. 8, no. 1, pp. 1–10.

Naughton, C, Drennan, J, & Lafferty, A 2014, 'Older people's perceptions of the term elder abuse and characteristics associated with a lower level of awareness', *Journal of Elder Abuse & Neglect*, vol. 26, no. 3, pp. 300–318.

Office for National Statistics 2015, 'Crime in England and Wales, year ending March 2015', *Statistical Bulletin*, Office for National Statistics.

Payne, BK 2010, 'Understanding elder sexual abuse and the criminal justice system's response: Comparison to elder physical abuse', *Justice Quarterly*, vol. 27, pp. 206–224.

Planty, M, Langton, L, Krebs, C, Berzofsky, M, & Smiley-McDonald, H 2013, *Female victims of sexual violence, 1994–2010*, Bureau of Justice Statistics, Office of Justice Programs, U.S. Department of Justice, Washington, DC.

Poulos, CA, & Sheridan, DJ 2008, 'Genital injuries in postmenopausal women after sexual assault', *Journal of Elder Abuse & Neglect*, vol. 20, pp. 323–335.

Ramsey-Klawsnik, H 1991, 'Elder sexual abuse: Preliminary findings', *Journal of Elder Abuse & Neglect*, vol. 3, no. 3, pp. 73–90.

Ramsey-Klawsnik, H, & Teaster, PB 2012, 'Sexual abuse happens in healthcare facilities: What can be done to prevent it?', *Generations*, vol. 36, pp. 53–59.

Ramsey-Klawsnik, H, Teaster, PB, Mendiondo, MS, Marcum, JL, & Abner, EL 2008, 'Sexual predators who target elders: Findings from the first national study of sexual abuse in care facilities', *Journal of Elder Abuse & Neglect*, vol. 20, pp. 353–376.

Roberto, KA 2016, 'The complexities of elder abuse', *American Psychologist*, vol. 71, pp. 302–311.

Roberto, KA, Brossoie, N, McPherson, M, Pulsifer, MB, & Brown, PN 2013, 'Violence against rural older women: Promoting community awareness and action', *Australasian Journal on Ageing*, vol. 32, no. 1, pp. 2–7.

Roberto, KA, & Teaster, PB 2005, 'Sexual abuse of vulnerable young and old women: A comparative analysis of circumstances and outcomes', *Violence against Women*, vol. 11, pp. 473–504.

Soares, J, Barros, H, Torres-Gonzales, F, Toannidi-Kapolou, E, Lamura, G, Lindert, J, . . . Stankūnas, M 2010, 'Abuse and health in Europe', Lithuanian University of Health Sciences Press. Retrieved from: www.hig.se/download/18.3984f2ed12e6a7b4c3580003555/ABUEL.pdf

Speck, PM, Hartig, MT, Likes, W, Bowdre, T, Carney, AY, Ekroos, RA, . . . Faugno, DK 2013, 'Analysis of possible sexual assault or abuse in a 67-year-old female with early Dementia post–brain attack', *Advanced Emergency Nursing Journal*, vol. 35, pp. 217–239.

Tarzia, L, Fetherstonghaugh, D, & Bauer, M 2012, 'Dementia, sexuality and consent in residential aged care facilities', *Journal of Medical Ethics*, vol. 38, pp. 609–613.

Teaster, PB, Ramsey-Klawsnik, H, Abner, EL, & Kim, S 2015, 'The sexual victimization of older women living in nursing homes', *Journal of Elder Abuse & Neglect*, vol. 27, no. 4/5, pp. 392–409.

Teaster, PB, & Roberto, KA 2003, 'Sexual abuse of older women living in nursing homes', *Journal of Gerontological Social Work*, vol. 40, pp. 105–119.

UN Women 2011, *Progress of the world's women 2011–2012: In pursuit of justice*, UN Women, New York.

Vierthaler, K 2008, 'Best practices for working with rape crisis centers to address elder sexual abuse', *Journal of Elder Abuse & Neglect*, vol. 20, pp. 306–322.

9

THE CHALLENGES IN REDUCING STIS WHILE FULFILLING AND ENHANCING THE SEXUAL RIGHTS OF OLDER PEOPLE

Graham Brown, Anthony Lyons, Sharron Hinchliff, and Pauline Crameri

Introduction

The cultural meanings, experiences of and education about sexually transmitted infections (STIs) among older people are markedly different from their younger counterparts. As described by Kirkman, Kenny and Fox (2013), while we cannot generalise completely, there are contexts regarding people older than 65 years of age that are important to consider. This population's cultural experiences of sexuality and sexual health have been "characterised by a letting go of traditional norms and exploration of new relationships," and particularly in Western countries, often referred to as the sexual revolution generation (Kirkman, Kenny & Fox 2013). Much of this group came of age post-contraceptive pill and pre-AIDS. Regardless of their individual sexual experiences, people older than 65 years are an important group to consider because they have lived through an era of increasing social acceptability of divorce, casual sex, sexual exploration and more recently online dating, but many have missed out on sex education and/or not been the target of STI prevention campaigns. These are quite unique challenges in the context of promoting sexual health and reducing the transmission and impact of STIs.

This chapter examines the evidence and developments in responding to STIs among older people, and the challenges in reducing STIs as well as fulfilling and enhancing the sexual rights of this group (as described in Chapter 2). We begin with a brief overview of the epidemiological, behavioural and social research concerning STIs among older people in Western countries, as this is where the majority of published research has been conducted. We then look at what we know about what works in STI prevention and discuss progress and challenges in policy, health and aged care services, health promotion, and research responding to STIs in older people. We end with a summary of opportunities to harness as we work towards the sexual health and rights of older people.

Epidemiological, behavioural and social research on STIs and older people

Over the past decade, diagnoses of STIs such as chlamydia, gonorrhoea and syphilis have increased significantly among older people in Western countries (Centers for Disease Control and Prevention 2014; Minichiello et al. 2012; Poynten, Grulich & Templeton 2013; The Kirby Institute 2015). While many Western countries are seeing rising rates of STIs among young adults (Centres for Disease Control and Prevention 2015; Public Health England 2016; The Kirby Institute 2015), this has somewhat masked other emerging epidemics. The published age categories for rate calculations across England, the U.S. and Australia vary, yet the trends are very similar. For example, in England the rates of chlamydia diagnoses in the 45–64 age group rose from 21.1 per 100,000 in 2010 to 39.7 per 100,000 in 2014, and in the 65+ age group from 1.5 per 100,000 in 2010 to 3.2 per 100,000 in 2014 (Public Health England 2016). In the U.S. rates of chlamydia diagnoses in the 55–64 age group rose from 9.7 per 100,000 in 2010 to 16.6 per 100,000 in 2014, and in the 65+ age group from 2.4 per 100,000 in 2010 to 3.2 per 100,000 in 2014 (Centres for Disease Control and Prevention 2015). Australia has seen similar increases in the 40+ age group, with rates of chlamydia diagnoses in the 55–64 age group rising from 16.4 per 100,000 in 2010 to 26.6 per 100,000 in 2014 (The Kirby Institute 2015). All three countries experienced similar increases in gonorrhoea and syphilis across these age groups, as well as sustained or increasing rates of HIV diagnoses, coupled with an ageing population of people previously diagnosed with HIV (Centers for Disease Control and Prevention 2014; Public Health England 2016; The Kirby Institute 2015).

Recent studies further indicate that older people who may have been exposed to an STI show low levels of testing. Studies in the U.S. found that only one out of three most-at-risk adults aged 50 years or older had accessed an STI test in the previous year (Schick et al. 2010), and that less than 20% of heterosexual participants aged 57–85 years had ever been tested for HIV (Harawa et al. 2011). Similarly low rates of testing have been found in Australia, with only 3.2% of men and 1.9% of women aged 60–69 years reporting an STI in the previous year (Grulich et al. 2014).

The majority of social, behavioural and knowledge research into sexual behaviour and STIs has focused on adolescents (Hendry et al. 2013). However, there have been some studies of or including older people. In Australia, a population-based study of people aged 16–69 years found those older than 60 had the lowest mean score for STI-related knowledge questions, such as how chlamydia, gonorrhoea and genital warts are transmitted, across all age groups (Grulich et al. 2014). Studies in the U.S. and Australia have also found that older adults were less likely than young people to use condoms (de Visser et al. 2014; Reece et al. 2010), including those whose behaviour may place them at increased risk of an STI (such as multiple or new partners) (Bateson et al. 2012; Schick et al. 2010)

An important factor to consider is that older age groups are more likely to be living with long-term health conditions that may contribute to sexual health problems. For example, menopause – which can sometimes cause vaginal dryness and thinning of vaginal tissues – erectile dysfunction associated with cardiovascular disease (CVD), diabetes, high blood pressure and a range of other conditions can increase problems in condom use (Department of Health 2013). Furthermore, due to a lack of pregnancy risk, and often previous long-term monogamous relationships, the motivations to use condoms may be absent in many instances (de Visser et al. 2014; Herbenick et al. 2010; Reece et al. 2010; Schick et al. 2010).

Thus, there is now substantial emerging evidence that the current cohort of older people may be at greater risk of STIs than previous older cohorts were, particularly in Western countries. Despite common misconceptions, older people are not asexual; therefore, it is important to recognise older people's sexual rights. The remaining sections of this chapter explore more closely issues of STI prevention, stigma and sexual rights of older people.

STI prevention, stigma and sexual rights

There has been substantial social research into the individual, interpersonal and structural impact of stigma in STI prevention, though much of this has focused on HIV (Hood & Friedman 2011; Mahajan et al. 2008; Sengupta et al. 2011; Stangl et al. 2013). Most studies have drawn on seminal theoretical work in stigma generally and in regard to sexual health and HIV (Goffman 1963; Link & Phelan 2001; Parker & Aggleton 2003).

The origins of stigma surrounding STIs are longstanding, multi-layered and embedded in the moralisation of sex throughout history (Hood & Friedman 2011). This often results in sexuality-related risks being judged more harshly by communities than other health risks (Conley et al. 2015), and are often exacerbated by other stigmas regarding race and class (Hood & Friedman 2011; Lichtenstein 2008; Parker & Aggleton 2003).

Stigma related to STIs can cause not only psychological suffering but also delays in seeking testing and treatment, as well as disclosure to sexual partners, which can all facilitate onward transmission (Hood & Friedman 2011). The stigma associated with STIs can be exacerbated for an older person who may be conscious of the stereotypes of older people as being asexual, and may therefore be embarrassed to even disclose that they are sexually active to health professionals. Stigma also impacts on the way STIs and sexual health are approached by communities, institutions (including aged care), and public health and medical agencies (Hood & Friedman 2011). To reduce STIs we need to challenge multiple forms of stigma, including both STI-related stigma and the stigma about older people's expression of sexuality. This means being committed to achieving the sexual rights of older people described in Chapter 2 as we strive to achieve the sexual rights of all people. While the full range of these sexual rights are clearly relevant, we will focus particularly on the following five:

- The right to equality and non-discrimination
- The right to the highest attainable standard of health including sexual health
- The right to enjoy the benefits of scientific progress and its application
- The right to information
- The right to education and the right to comprehensive sexuality education

Evidence of what works in STI prevention

A major part of meeting older people's right to information and comprehensive education, and equitable access to the latest sexual health care, is to ensure available age-appropriate education and support for STI prevention. The majority of systematic literature reviews on effective STI prevention are focused on young people and young adults (e.g. see Brown et al. 2013; Kang, Skinner & Usherwood 2010; Lazarus et al. 2010) or groups most at risk of HIV (Brown et al. 2015). Consistent with broader health promotion principles (WHO 1986), these reviews agree that programs are most effective in increasing protective behaviours for STIs when they:

- target multiple components of people's lives, the contexts in which they live, and address multiple domains across interpersonal, social and structural levels;
- are skills-based, self-efficacy-based and motivation-based programs and explicitly based on recognised behavioural and social theories;
- are a part of a package of sexual health interventions operating across different health promotion levels at the individual, group, community and structural or system level; and
- are in a sexual rights and enabling policy environment that supports integrated primary care, community and media strategies (Brown et al. 2013).

Despite this evidence, most STI policies and programs focus on risk, negative outcomes and deficits rather than strategies embedded in the reality of the sexual and social lives, relationships and sexual rights of their target populations (Brown et al. 2013).

Although at face value these broad findings may seem transferable to all STI prevention programs regardless of population group, we know very little about the transferability of STI programs aimed at young adults to older adults, or the broader structural and policy-level conditions needed to support them. However, the multiple-level approach to STI prevention and health promotion underpinning these recommendations (i.e. responding at the policy level, clinical health services level and the community level) provides a useful framework to discuss the progress and challenges of preventing STIs among older people and illustrates the relationship with sexual rights outlined earlier.

Progress and challenges in responding to STIs in older people

Drawing on current evidence and health promotion theory, in this section we discuss developments and issues in STI prevention and achieving the above sexual rights among older people with regard to: (1) policy-level responses and an enabling environment; (2) health services (primary care and sexual health); (3) community health promotion; and (4) social and epidemiological research to support an evidence-based holistic response.

An enabling policy-level response

The Ottawa Charter for Health Promotion (WHO 1986) identified health policy responses and an enabling environment as key components in the improvement of health. In the promotion of sexual health this includes programs, services and strategies working in, and challenging, taboo areas. For example, the HIV response in Western countries like Australia entailed more than changes in behaviour; they also focused on reforming laws, policies, and health and social services; ensuring affected community participation in quality research; ensuring a human-rights-based response; and challenging prejudice, ideology and dogma as barriers to effective health promotion (Brown et al. 2014).

Policies that support or guide the response to STIs impact on the achievement of the five sexual rights identified previously. Although many countries do not have national STI or sexual health policies, those that do identify young people as the primary or only priority (Hendry et al. 2013; Kirkman, Kenny & Fox 2013). The majority of STI diagnoses are amongst younger adults (Centers for Disease Control and Prevention 2014; Public Health England 2016; The Kirby Institute 2015), and so it makes sense to focus the policy and program investment to those groups. However, the social, behavioural and epidemiological changes over the past few decades are substantial, and STIs among older people is an emerging epidemic in need of attention. The nuanced needs of older people should be addressed in terms of STI education as well as testing and treatment (Schick et al. 2010); however, few policy structures or responses meet the needs of older adults (Gott 2005; MacDonald et al. 2015). To illustrate the challenges, we look at recent policy responses in three developed countries: Australia, UK and US.

Australia has developed a suite of strategies to "promote multi-level, integrated and comprehensive health promotion programs" in response to blood-borne viruses and STIs (Australian Government 2014). Although the 2014–2017 National STI Strategy argues for sex education to be integrated within a broader range of health promotion activities, the STI Strategy does not discuss education for individuals outside of priority populations, and engagement opportunities such as new media are only discussed in the context of the strategy's first priority: young people. A review by Kirkman, Kenny and Fox (2013) of earlier strategies and policy documents across Australian federal, state and territory governments also found a focus on risk, not well-being, in relation to sexual health, and an emphasis on adolescents, young adults and reproduction, which excluded older people.

The 'Framework for Sexual Health Improvement in England' (Department of Health 2013) discusses sexual health across the lifespan. Although the most detailed sections relate to young people and young adults, encouragingly, people aged over 50 are specifically identified. The framework identifies particular health implications of

STIs in older populations and also older people living with HIV. However, despite explicitly discussing people over 50, the framework has made little mention of concrete actions except for older adults living with undiagnosed HIV.

Like many countries, the US has achieved a National HIV Strategy, but despite conducting consultations regarding a national response to STIs (Centers for Disease Control and Prevention 2010) – which included advice to respond to STIs across the lifespan and had concerted advocacy calling for a coordinated approach to STIs (Swartzendruber & Zenilman 2010) – there has not yet been consensus on a national sexual health and STI prevention framework. However, STIs were included as one of the 42 topic areas within the U.S. Office of Disease Prevention and Health Promotion Healthy People 2020 (launched in 2010), a set of 10-year national goals and objectives for improving population health. While the discussion for the topic area highlights the importance of the sexual health of older people, all the measurable objectives relate to the age groups 15–24 or 15–44 years (Office of Disease Prevention and Health Promotion 2016).

There is often recognition in the aforementioned policy documents about the need to create an enabling environment for the prevention of STIs; however, they most commonly focus on responding to the education needs of young people and rarely articulate action for structural reform in funding priorities, health services or broader cultural change in regard to older population groups. Epidemiological patterns and limited resources for sexual health promotion are appropriately major factors driving these priorities; it is likely they are not the only factors. The impact of stigma on social and health policy has been well identified (Hatzenbuehler, Phelan & Link 2013; Kirkman, Kenny & Fox 2013; Parker & Aggleton 2003), and in this instance we have multiple intersecting forms of stigma, including stigma of sexuality in general, older people's sexuality in particular (Hinchliff, Gott & Ingleton 2010; Hood & Friedman 2011), and stigma related to STIs and sexual risk (Conley et al. 2015), as well as the political difficulties of challenging long-held social and cultural taboos (Link & Phelan 2001). These can accumulate and result in the devaluing of the sexual health of older people.

Health services (primary care, aged care and sexual health services)

The reorientation of health services to meet the needs of changing communities was also identified by the Ottawa Charter (WHO 1986) as a key component in the improvement of health. This is no less central in the reduction of STIs and the achievement of sexual rights (such as the right to the highest attainable standard of health, including sexual health, and the right to enjoy the benefits of scientific progress and its application, as described earlier and in Chapter 2) where timely, voluntary and respectful testing and treatment of STIs is critical.

When the policy focus excludes or de-emphasises the importance of STIs among older people (as described above), this can impact not only on the investment in health services but also on the training, education and attitudes amongst health and aged care professionals and providers. For example, as argued by Kirkman, Kenny and Fox (2013), the education of health professionals has rarely included older people's sexual health. This leads to fewer sexual histories being taken and fewer STI tests being performed, and thus surveillance data do not reflect actual prevalence of infections across all age groups, and consequently are less likely to be acknowledged or prioritised in the education of health and aged care professionals.

As described earlier in this chapter, there are unique factors to consider around the sexual health of older people, which are related to the management and impact of co-morbidities as well as generational and social assumptions and stereotypes. Hinchliff and Gott (2011) conducted a systematic review of literature concerning help-seeking for, and doctor-patient interactions about, sexual health problems in older people. Some of the barriers identified by Hinchliff and Gott (2011) included psychosocial factors for the patient (such as assuming that sexual changes were a 'normal' part of ageing) and for the physician (such as assuming that sex was less important to older patients). The review also found, as with other population groups, that older people were more likely to seek help if their doctor had previously asked about sexual functioning or sexuality during a previous routine visit. However, physicians tended not to be proactive in sexual health management and generally had limited knowledge of later-life sexuality issues. Despite the disinclination to discuss sexual health issues with certain patients, Grant and Ragsdale (2008) found that most physicians thought they were adequately prepared for such discussions.

There have been consistent findings in literature concerning physicians bringing societal age, gender and sexuality biases to their perceptions regarding which patients they believe are sexually active and the sexual health needs of older people and the influence this has on their communication about sexual health (Bitzer 2011; Gott, Hinchliff & Galena 2004; Grant & Ragsdale 2008; Maes & Louis 2011; Slinkard & Kazer 2011). The barriers that both the older patient and the health professional bring to any discussion about sexual health impacts the quality of the consultation (Bitzer 2011; Slinkard & Kazer 2011). Past interactions with health providers regarding sexuality, relationships and sexual health impact on the ability of older people to communicate with health providers (Gott & Hinchliff 2003; Hughes 2013) and can in effect either give older people a sense of "permission" to raise sexual health issues or deter them from seeking help (Hinchliff & Gott 2011). When health services or aged care providers avoid the topic of sexuality and sexual function, they reinforce assumptions within their patients that they either should not have sexual concerns or should not raise them.

It is essential that health services and practitioners working with older people are attentive to the diverse sexual health needs of older people, including pleasure, difficulties, and concerns.

Creating a climate and patient-practitioner relationship in which sexual behaviour and function can be discussed supports not only STI diagnoses and treatment but also the fulfilment of sexual rights and to achieve general wellbeing (Barrett 2011; Gott, Hinchliff & Galena 2004; Lottes 2013; Schick et al. 2010).

Community health promotion

Community sexual health promotion campaigns are an important part of contributing to sexual rights, particularly the right to information and the right to education and comprehensive sexuality education as described earlier and in Chapter 2. However, community health promotion for the prevention of STIs is often limited to occasional paid advertising campaigns, and these overwhelmingly focus on young people or young adults with an emphasis on condom use, risk and negative outcomes, including STIs and unplanned pregnancy (Hendry et al. 2013; Kirkman, Kenny & Fox 2013). As described earlier, paid advertising campaigns are only one component of a multi-level integrated community health promotion approach to preventing STIs (Brown et al. 2013).

There have been calls for community health promotion to focus on older people, STIs, condom use and testing (Kirkman, Kenny & Fox 2013; Schick et al. 2010). One of the few literature reviews regarding STI prevention interventions for older people (MacDonald et al. 2015) involved a review of studies trialling condom promotion strategies for people aged 40+, updating an earlier review by (Davis & Zanjani 2012). It found few studies (five interventions) and all were conducted in the U.S., with four focusing on HIV prevention for ethnic minority men. The review found mixed results, with little evidence that current strategies (as few as they are) are effective, with only one intervention showing a significant effect. The authors highlighted that previous reviews of condom promotion interventions generally found that interventions were reliant on a number of population-specific factors to be effective, including age, gender and sexual orientation (MacDonald et al. 2015). Other studies highlighted that there are significant differences in the promotion of condoms for older people, such as when there is no risk of conception or there may be a higher proportion with difficulties using condoms that are quite different from young audiences (Schick et al. 2010). This suggests that the transferability of evidence from specific interventions between population groups is highly problematic.

The emphasis of current campaigns on adolescents and young adults has an influence on perceptions of sexual behaviour and STIs among older people. The lack of a sustained visible response for older people may reinforce assumptions that only younger adults are sexually active and that STIs are the fault and privilege of 'reckless immoral youth'. As argued by Hood and Friedman (2011), the implicit message is that those who acquire STIs should have the power and autonomy to control their interpersonal relationships and sexual networks – a message that also ignores the broader sociocultural determinants that influence sexual partnering, risk and STI acquisition.

Public health has a history of inadvertently reinforcing stigma and barriers in its response to STIs. As argued by Hood and Friedman (2011), STI prevention campaigns have in the past employed stigmatising messaging and images, and even scare tactics, to motivate people to adopt risk-reduction behaviours. While the promotion of sexual health has progressed over the past few decades, it is important to recognise that many people over 65 lived through some of the more stigmatising campaigns and strategies in STI and HIV prevention. We need to ensure that current STI strategies, even by omission, do not inadvertently reinforce stereotypes and undermine the promotion of sexual health and sexual rights for older people.

It is important to recognise, however, that most STI campaigns do not find their way into the scientific literature and indeed are not evidence-based. Encouragingly, over the past five years there have been more examples of investment in campaigns specifically targeting sexual health and STIs among older people, including online campaigns, such as the U.S. (e.g. SaferSex4Seniors.org in 2012), Australia (www.fpnsw.org.au/littleblackdress in 2012) and UK (www.fpa.org.uk/campaignsandadvocacy/sexualhealthweek/stisandsafersexover50 in 2010). Although strongly sex positive, these campaigns have generally been small ad-hoc responses endeavouring to make a contribution to an ongoing gap, and have needed to be as much about raising awareness of older people's sexuality as they have about sexual health.

There is evidence that some older people find that the internet provides a safe platform to meet sexual partners, access information, enhance their sexual knowledge and avoid stigma (Alterovitz & Mendelsohn 2013; Bateson et al. 2012), thus providing emerging new opportunities for effective engagement with this population. Engagement with these opportunities will require a deeper understanding of how older people utilise these online spaces and not presuming the same patterns as younger online participants. This issue and the missed opportunities for sexual health promotion for older people is discussed further in Chapter 11.

An important tenet of the Ottawa Health Promotion Charter and the sexual rights described in Chapter 2 is the recognition that communities are not passive recipients of sexual health promotion. Experience from across the sexual health and HIV fields has shown that harnessing the resilience, innovation and participation of communities has been central to effective responses (Brown et al. 2014). People over 65 oversaw some of the largest international movements in sexual liberation. As described in Chapter 2, responding to sexual rights and preventing STIs in older people will mean working with, rather than intervening on, our older communities.

Social, epidemiological and policy research

Quality social and epidemiological research is important not only for guiding STI prevention but also for achieving sexual rights. The right to the benefits of scientific progress and its application and the right to information (as described earlier and in Chapter 2) includes research into what works to reduce STIs through policies, health services and health promotion strategies, although, as mentioned earlier, is largely aimed at young people (Hendry et al. 2013; Kirkman, Kenny & Fox 2013). This includes research into the use of social media for sexual health promotion.

We need a health response based on accurate and relevant research across population groups and not based on assumptions that research with young people will be transferable to the sexual health needs of older people. We also need to monitor the unintended outcomes of current STI prevention strategies on non-priority target groups, for example, the unintended stigmatising or de-prioritising of sexual health concerns in older people.

It is a step in the right direction that there has been an increase in social and epidemiological research into the sexual health needs and experiences of older people (Hinchliff & Gott 2011; MacDonald et al. 2015; Minichiello et al. 2012; Nash et al. 2015). What is needed now is further research into effective sexual health promotion for older people, as well as an evaluation of integrated responses across age groups. However, this is not to say that responses are aimless without targeted research. There are basic principles of sexual health rights and health promotion that can guide responses as well as the targeting of research in the meantime.

Conclusion

All people regardless of age need the highest level of health and wellbeing in relation to their sexuality, and this includes up-to-date information about STIs. Older people have the right to access comprehensive sexuality education, health promotion and sexual health services based on epidemiology and social research relevant to their age group. This chapter has explored the challenges and opportunities for the prevention of STIs in older people through a multi-level approach involving policy, health and aged care services, community health promotion and research. We have highlighted the relationship between the prevention of STIs in older people and the achievement of sexual health and rights, in particular: the right to equality and non-discrimination; the right to the highest attainable standard of health, including sexual health; the right to enjoy the benefits of scientific progress and its application; the right to information; and the right to education and comprehensive sexuality education. In order to make steps towards attaining these rights, we emphasise the following opportunities and recommendations:

- Policy – harness the increasing community and political engagement in the health and rights of older people to live well, the participation of older people in political advocacy, and the emerging evidence on the sexual health needs of older people. These factors together may help to make significant inroads to a policy environment that enables an effective response to the sexual rights of older people. However, this will require leadership not only across health and aged care services, community health promotion and research, but will also need to be incorporated into the advocacy for older people's health generally.
- Health services – recognise the social and cultural differences of people aged 65 years or older compared to previous generations. Acknowledging that many older people engage in sex, not making assumptions about their sexual lives, and raising the issue about sexual function and relationships with older people may give permission or confidence for them to raise discussions about sexual health more broadly and enhance communication between clinician and patient.

- Community health promotion – older people are not passive recipients of community health promotion. We have an opportunity to draw on the community resilience and mobilisation experiences of older people, and their engagement with new technologies and relationship opportunities, to develop relevant, engaging and evidence-based community health programmes. However, this needs to be complemented by strategies with other population groups that do not reinforce stereotypes.
- Research – enhance the current social and epidemiological research to guide and support an effective response to STIs in older people. At the same time, we also have an opportunity to enhance the evaluation of current initiatives to build a stronger evidence base of effective sexual health promotion for older people.

The most effective way to prevent the transmission of STIs would be to take a holistic approach based on these recommendations. The prevention of STIs, the promotion of sexual health, and the achievement of sexual rights are intertwined. Responding to STIs among older people will not be tackled through occasional or ad-hoc health promotion strategies. What is required is an integrated and sustained response across policy, health and aged care services, community health promotion and research.

References

Alterovitz, SSR & Mendelsohn, GA 2013, 'Relationship goals of middle-aged, young-old, and old-old internet daters: An analysis of online personal ads', *Journal of Aging Studies*, vol. 27, no. 2, pp. 159–165.

Australian Government 2014, *National STI strategy 2014–2017*, Commonwealth Government of Australia, Canberra.

Barrett, CM 2011, 'Auditing organisational capacity to promote the sexual health of older people', *Sensoria: A Journal of Mind, Brain & Culture*, vol. 7, no. 1, pp. 31–36.

Bateson, DJ, Weisberg, E, McCaffery, KJ & Luscombe, GM 2012, 'When online becomes offline: Attitudes to safer sex practices in older and younger women using an Australian internet dating service', *Sexual Health*, vol. 9, pp. 152–159.

Bitzer, J 2011, 'Promoting the sexual health of the older couple', *Aging Health*, vol. 7, no. 5, pp. 681–693.

Brown, G, Croy, S, Johnston, K, Pitts, M & Lewis, V 2013, *Rapid review: Reducing sexually transmissible infections in young people*, Australian Institute for Primary Care & Ageing (AIPCA) and Australian Research Centre in Sex, Health & Society (ARCSHS), La Trobe University, Melbourne, Australia.

Brown, G, O'Donnell, D, Crooks, L & Lake, R 2014, 'Mobilisation, politics, investment and constant adaptation: Lessons from the Australian health-promotion response to HIV', *Health Promotion Journal of Australia*, vol. 25, pp. 35–41.

Brown, G, Reeders, D, Dowsett, GW, Ellard, J, Carman, M, Hendry, N & Wallace, J 2015, 'Investigating combination HIV prevention: Isolated interventions or complex system', *Journal of the International AIDS Society*, vol. 18, no. 1, pp. 204–299

Centers for Disease Control and Prevention 2010, *A public health approach for advancing sexual health in the United States: Rationale and options for implementation, meeting report of an external consultation*, Atlanta, Georgia, <www.cdc.gov/sexualhealth/docs/SexualHealthReport-2011-508.pdf>.

C:\Users\smitchell\Desktop\My Titles\Barrett 15031-1180\02 Barrett CE files\15031-1180-Ref Mismatch Report.docx - LStERROR_34——— 2014, *Sexually transmitted disease surveillance 2013*, Department of Health and Human Services, Atlanta, US.

——— 2015, *Sexually transmitted disease surveillance 2014*, U.S. Department of Health and Human Services, Atlanta, <www.cdc.gov/std/stats/default.htm>.

Conley, TD, Moors, AC, Matsick, JL & Ziegler, A 2015, 'Sexuality-related risks are judged more harshly than comparable health risks', *International Journal of Sexual Health*, vol. 27, no. 4, pp. 508–521.

Davis, T & Zanjani, F 2012, 'Prevention of HIV among older adults: A literature review and recommendations for future research', *Journal of Aging and Health*, vol. 24, no. 8, pp. 1399–1420.

Department of Health 2013, *A framework for sexual health improvement in England*, Government of England, London, UK, viewed 15 March 2013, <www.dh.gsi.gov.uk/mandate>.

de Visser, RO, Badcock, PB, Rissel, C, Richters, J, Smith, AM, Grulich, AE & Simpson, JM 2014, 'Safer sex and condom use: Findings from the second Australian study of health and relationships', *Sexual Health*, vol. 11, no. 5, pp. 495–504.

Goffman, E 1963, *Stigma: Notes on the management of spoiled identity*, Prentice-Hall, Englewood Cliffs.

Gott, M 2005, 'Are older people at risk of sexually transmitted infections? A new look at the evidence', *Reviews in Clinical Gerontology*, vol. 14, pp. 5–13.

Gott, M & Hinchliff, S 2003, 'Barriers to seeking treatment for sexual problems in primary care: A qualitative study with older people', *Family Practice*, vol. 20, no. 6, pp. 690–695.

Gott, M, Hinchliff, S & Galena, E 2004, 'General practitioner attitudes to discussing sexual health issues with older people', *Social Science and Medicine*, vol. 58, pp. 2093–2103.

Grant, K & Ragsdale, K 2008, 'Sex and the "recently single": Perceptions of sexuality and HIV risk among mature women and primary care physicians', *Culture, Health & Sexuality*, vol. 10, no. 5, pp. 495–511.

Grulich, AE, de Visser, RO, Badcock, PB, Smith, AM, Richters, J, Rissel, C & Simpson, JM 2014, 'Knowledge about and experience of sexually transmissible infections in a representative sample of adults: The second Australian study of health and relationships', *Sexual Health*, vol. 11, no. 5, pp. 481–494.

Harawa, NT, Leng, M, Kim, J & Cunningham, WE 2011, 'Racial/ethnic and gender differences among older adults in nonmonogamous partnerships, time spent single, and HIV testing', *Sexually Transmitted Diseases*, vol. 38, no. 12, pp. 1110–1117.

Hatzenbuehler, ML, Phelan, JC & Link, BG 2013, 'Stigma as a fundamental cause of population health inequalities', *American Journal of Public Health*, vol. 103, no. 5, pp. 813–821.

Hendry, N, Brown, G, Johnston, K & Dowsett, G 2013, *Beyond high school: What do we know about young adults' social and sexual contexts?*, Australian Research Centre in Sex, Health and Society, La Trobe University, Melbourne, Australia.

Herbenick, D, Reece, M, Schick, V, Sanders, SA, Dodge, B & Fortenberry, DJ 2010, 'Sexual behavior in the United States: Results from a national probability sample of men and women ages 14–94', *Journal of Sexual Medicine*, vol. 7, no. Supplement 5, pp. 255–265.

Hinchliff, S & Gott, M 2011, 'Seeking medical help for sexual concerns in mid- and later life: A review of the literature', *Journal of Sex Research*, vol. 48, no. 2–3, pp. 106–117.

Hinchliff, S, Gott, M & Ingleton, C 2010, 'Sex, menopause and social context: A qualitative study with heterosexual women', *Journal of Health Psychology*, vol. 15, no. 5, pp. 724–733.

Hood, JE & Friedman, AL 2011, 'Unveiling the hidden epidemic: A review of stigma associated with sexually transmissible infections', *Sexual Health*, vol. 8, no. 2, pp. 159–170.

Hughes, AK 2013, 'Mid-to-late-life women and sexual health: Communication with health care providers', *Family Medicine*, vol. 45, no. 4, pp. 252–256.

Kang, M, Skinner, R & Usherwood, T 2010, 'Interventions for young people in Australia to reduce HIV and sexually transmissible infections: A systematic review', *Sexual Health*, vol. 7, no. 2, pp. 107–128.

The Kirby Institute 2015, *HIV, viral hepatitis and sexually transmissible infections in Australia annual surveillance report 2015*, Sydney, NSW.

Kirkman, L, Kenny, A & Fox, C 2013, 'Evidence of absence: Midlife and older adult sexual health policy in Australia', *Sexuality Research and Social Policy*, vol. 10, no. 2, pp. 135–148.

Lazarus, JV, Sihvonen-Riemenschneider, H, Laukamm-Josten, U, Wong, F & Liljestrand, J 2010, 'Systematic review of interventions to prevent the spread of sexually transmitted infections, including HIV, among young people in Europe', *Croatian Medical Journal*, vol. 51, no. 1, pp. 74–84.

Lichtenstein, B 2008, '"Exemplary elders": Stigma, stereotypes and sexual transmitted infections among older African Americans', *Current Sociology*, vol. 56, no. 1, pp. 99–114.

Link, BG & Phelan, JC 2001, 'Conceptualizing stigma', *Annual review of Sociology*, vol. 27, no. 1, pp. 363–385.

Lottes, IL 2013, 'Sexual rights: Meanings, controversies, and sexual health promotion', *The Journal of Sex Research*, vol. 50, no. 3–4, pp. 367–391.

MacDonald, J, Lorimer, K, Knussen, C & Flowers, P 2015, 'Interventions to increase condom use among middle-aged and older adults: A systematic review of theoretical bases, behaviour change techniques, modes of delivery and treatment fidelity', *Journal of Health Psychology*, vol. 21, no. 11, pp. 2477–2492.

Maes, CA & Louis, M 2011, 'Nurse Practitioners' Sexual History-Taking Practices with Adults 50 and Older. *The Journal for Nurse Practitioners*, vol. 7, no. 3, pp. 216–222.

Mahajan, AP, Sayles, JN, Patel, VA, Remien, RH, Ortiz, D, Szekeres, G & Coates, TJ 2008, 'Stigma in the HIV/AIDS epidemic: A review of the literature and recommendations for the way forward', *AIDS (London, England)*, vol. 22, no. Supplement 2, p. S67.

Minichiello, V, Rahman, S, Hawkes, G & Pitts, M 2012, 'STI epidemiology in the global older population: Emerging challenges', *Perspectives in Public Health*, vol. 132, no. 4, pp. 178–181.

Nash, P, Willis, P, Tales, A & Cryer, T 2015, 'Sexual health and sexual activity in later life', *Reviews in Clinical Gerontology*, vol. 25, no. 1, pp. 22–30.

Office of Disease Prevention and Health Promotion 2016, *2020 Topics & objectives: Sexually transmitted diseases*, Office of Disease Prevention and Health Promotion, Altanta, USA, viewed 1 March 2016, <www.healthypeople.gov/2020/topics-objectives/topic/sexually-transmitted-diseases>.

Parker, R & Aggleton, P 2003, 'HIV and AIDS-related stigma and discrimination: A conceptual framework and implications for action', *Social Science & Medicine*, vol. 57, no. 1, pp. 13–24.

Poynten, IM, Grulich, AE & Templeton, DJ 2013, 'Sexually transmitted infections in older populations', *Current Opinion in Infectious Diseases*, vol. 26, no. 1, pp. 80–85.

Public Health England 2016, *Sexually transmitted infections (STIs): Annual data tables*, England, viewed 1 March 2014, <www.gov.uk/government/statistics/sexually-transmitted-infections-stis-annual-data-tables>.

Reece, M, Herbenick, D, Schick, V, Sanders, SA, Dodge, B & Fortenberry, DJ 2010, 'Condom use rates in a national probability sample of males and females ages 14 to 94 in the United States', *Journal of Sexual Medicine*, vol. 7, no. Supplement 5, pp. 266–276.

Schick, V, Herbenick, D, Reece, M, Sanders, SA, Dodge, B, Middlestadt, SE & Fortenberry, DJ 2010, 'Sexual behaviors, condom use, and sexual health of Americans over 50: Implications for sexual health promotion for older adults', *Journal of Sexual Medicine*, vol. 7, no. Supplement 5, pp. 315–329.

Sengupta, S, Banks, B, Sheps, CG, Jonas, D, Miles, MS & Smith, GC 2011, 'HIV interventions to reduce HIV/AIDS stigma: A systematic review', *Aids Behavior*, vol. 15, no. 6, pp. 1075–1087.

Slinkard, MS & Kazer, MW 2011, 'Older adults and HIV and STI screening: The patient perspective', *Geriatric Nursing*, vol. 32, no. 5, pp. 341–349.

Stangl, AL, Lloyd, JK, Brady, LM, Holland, CE & Baral, S 2013, 'A systematic review of interventions to reduce HIV-related stigma and discrimination from 2002 to 2013: How far have we come?', *Journal of the International AIDS Society*, vol. 16, no. 3, Supplement 2, p. 18734.

Swartzendruber, A & Zenilman, JM 2010, 'A national strategy to improve sexual health', *JAMA*, vol. 304, no. 9, pp. 1005–1006.

WHO 1986, *Ottawa charter for health promotion*, WHO/HPR/HEP/95.1, World Health Organisation, Geneva, <www.who.int/healthpromotion/conferences/previous/ottawa/en/index4.html>.

10

CHALLENGING THE 'VIAGRIZATION' OF HETEROSEXUALITY AND AGEING

Catherine Barrett, Emily Wentzell, and Raffaella Ferrero Camoletto

Introduction

Viagra was developed by Pfizer in 1998 and is one of their top-selling drugs, with $2 billion worldwide revenue in 2012 alone (Trenton 2013). Pfizer reports that there are around 30 million men in the U.S. with 'erectile dysfunction' and that more than 23 million men have been prescribed Viagra (Pfizer 2016). It works by increasing blood flow to the penis and was initially manufactured for older men with erectile difficulties related to medical problems (Lexchin 2006). However, after Viagra's release, Pfizer marketed the drug to a broader cohort of men who are interested in harder, longer-lasting erections, shifting the focus from therapeutic use (making erection possible) to recreational and lifestyle use (enhancing erectile quality) (Loe 2004a; Baglia 2005; Lexchin 2006).

Viagra and its competitors have been heralded as a therapeutic revolution, enabling men to overcome the fear and shame related to erectile dysfunction (Pantalone et al. 2008). These drugs enable men to continue to conform to stereotypical norms of masculinity in which penetrative vaginal sex is key (Tiefer 1986, 1994; Connell & Messerschmidt 2005). Viagra is also credited with promoting awareness of older men's sexuality. It could be argued that older men taking Viagra are asserting their right to enjoy the benefits of scientific progress and their right to achieve the highest attainable level of sexual health and well-being. However, this view is somewhat simplistic. As Tiefer (1994) suggests, there has been a 'viagrization' of older men's sexuality arising from vascular discourses that reframe age-related erectile decline (which we will refer to as ARED) as erectile 'dysfunction' (which is often referred to as ED), and encourage what Marshall (2010, 2012) calls 'virility surveillance'.

This reframing has been driven by the profit motives of pharmaceutical companies (Conrad & Leiter 2004). It capitalises on ageist views of bodily aging as pathology to be cured (Lamb 2014) and represents the move to maintain youthful standards of sexual function and attractiveness as indicators of 'successful' ageing (Gott 2004, 2006; Marshall 2011). All heterosexual men are assumed to desire sex and to hope to live out conventional forms of masculinity through their sexual behaviour (Loe 2001, 2004a; Tiefer 1986, 1994). In such discourses women are absent – except for a limited focus on their assumed life-long desire for vaginal penetration and a few studies exploring women's accounts of ED drugs' social impacts on their lives (e.g. Potts et al. 2003, 2004; Loe 2004b).

In this chapter we challenge phallocentric, ageist discourses about older people's sexuality by critiquing the idea that sexual rights in older age are synonymous with the right to access medical intervention to continue youthful and normative forms of sexuality. Instead, we argue that older people's right to sexuality is better served by enabling access to comprehensive, age-appropriate sexuality education that supports diverse and changing sexual expression throughout later life and is grounded in sexuality-positive approaches. We begin by tracing the emergence of phallocentric discourses and their influence on sexuality and ageing. We present the perspectives of medical specialists to examine how decisions about 'the legitimate patient' are made, showing how understanding access to treatment for ARED as the cornerstone of seniors' right to sexuality actually limits their sexual expression.

We then examine how Viagra has affected older women's sexuality, especially in terms of gendered power imbalances. We emphasise the importance of addressing psychological and relationship factors that impact on erectile function and partner interest in sex. The focus is then expanded to explore the ways in which a cultural perspective enables masculinity, sexuality and Viagra to be understood differently. This broad cultural lens is then utilised to present an approach to comprehensive sexuality education for older people.

The chapter focuses on Viagra (rather than sexuopharmaceuticals more broadly) and heterosexuality because of the literature available. For example, very little research exists on the important issue of same-sex-attracted older people's experiences of sexual function change and sexual health medicine (e.g. Jones & Pugh 2005; Slevin & Linneman 2010; Lodge & Umberson 2013). The public health literature that does exist on gay men and Viagra use reproduces stereotypes of gay sexuality as deviant by focusing on ED drug use in relationship to sexually transmissible infections rather than on sexual experience or satisfaction (Wentzell 2011).

Viagrization of older men's sexuality

Change in sexual function was previously considered an inevitable part of ageing (Katz & Marshall 2003) to which people were expected to adjust gracefully (Marshall 2011). Bodily ageing is now viewed as a pathology to be cured (Lamb 2017) rather than embraced, and theories of 'Successful Ageing' and 'Active Ageing' require that we strive to be ageless (Katz 2001; Lamb 2015). The push to agelessness has influenced the ways sexuality is conceptualised and the importance attributed to it. Significant emphasis is now placed on maintaining youthful standards of sexual function and attractiveness, and assumptions about biology are reworked to reflect this view (Marshall 2011). Sexuality is now an important part of the expectation of healthy, active ageing, and 'sexiness' is a way of distinguishing oneself as not old (Marshall 2011). In addition, sex is now considered a healthy and necessary component of successful ageing (Katz & Marshall, 2003; Calasanti & King 2005).

These expectations of sexuality and ageing create new sites of anxiety (Marshall 2011) that are recognised by pharmaceutical companies, who position themselves and their products to respond. This dynamic is particularly evident in the rebranding of ARED as ED, a physical disease requiring medical intervention (Riska 2003). Viagra offers a cure for something that was previously considered 'normal' in old age (Gross & Blundo 2005; Lamb 2015).

Lexchin (2006) suggests that 'disease mongering' by pharmaceutical companies ignores research showing strong associations between ED and psychological factors, and works to convince men that Viagra is the first choice for therapy for any degree of ED regardless of the cause. Such medications to make us 'better than well' need to be marketed as treatments for newly discovered disorders to ensure that physicians will prescribe them and to ensure they sell (Caplan & Elliot 2004). But medical specialists are also questioning Viagra as a 'magic bullet' and the consumerist notion that older men have the right to access this technology (Ferrero Camoletto et al. 2015; Ferrero Camoletto & Bertone 2017).

Challenging the 'magic bullet': the legitimate patient

Ferrero Camoletto and others (2015, 2017) conducted research in Italy to explore the concept of the 'legitimate patient,' or how decisions were made about who was entitled to Viagra prescription. The research involved interviews with 19 specialists in male sexual health (urologists, endocrinologists, sexologists, sexual counsellors) in different publicly funded health services. Specialists reported that patients had the right to 'active' and 'positive' ageing, as well as a duty to take care of their health across the lifespan by adopting a healthy and active lifestyle. In this context, specialists considered it legitimate for middle-aged and older men to seek assistance to maintain active sexual lives. However, issues were raised about the costs and who was entitled to access such treatment. For example, one specialist questioned whether he should invest his available budget on two patients in need of a radical cystectomy or one patient who was 'over 80, maybe with a 30 years younger partner, [who] desires a performance no longer adequate to biological age'.

This raises interesting questions about the prescription of Viagra for older men. What is an adequate sexual performance for older men? Who decides? When is pharma-mediated sexual functioning a sexual right for older men? Some specialists described feeling the need to contain and re-orient towards reality those they described as 'dirty old men' (Walz 2002) who chased an impossible return to youth. As one specialist reflected:

The point is that these drugs, and the campaigns and media too, make it impossible for the patient to get old any more. . . . Therefore it becomes a disease; in the past, without the drug, people came to terms with it.

The specialists had an active role in reproducing and questioning the notions of sexuality, masculinity and ageing conveyed by the marketing of medications like Viagra. Their discourses showed problematization of the ideal of a forever sexually functional man as the enactment of an always-ready and always-in-control hypermasculinity.

The criterion that specialists used to inform their treatment decisions was actually a moral boundary. They believed that deserving patients sought to repair sexual functioning within stable relationships, whereas improper ED drug seekers hoped for a second youth to be spent with younger partners within recreational or exchange-based relationships. As one specialist reported:

Taking a step back into the past, the man of a certain age who lived in his family with the idea of getting older was content with the old wife as a companion and so on; he smoothly dragged himself towards old age, and . . . boom! There was a shock because he could use this drug giving him the possibility to get back to the game again [laughing].

The specialists' reactions to the demands of older patients were plural and sometimes ambivalent, showing a lack of consensus. A crucial dimension was a tendency to weave biological and moral timing into decisions about the legitimate patient. As one specialist stated:

I am not here to make a 60 year old person go back to 20. . . . You should always interpret the evolution of Mother Earth, ok, and sexuality should be comparable to what should be right for each phase of life.

This critical position demonstrates the tension between the access to pharmacological innovations and supporting older men to adjust to age-related changes. It demonstrates the power of medical gatekeepers in determining what constitutes wellbeing. In so doing the specialists questioned the claim for older men's new sexual rights made available by the advent of Viagra: on the contrary, they criticised what they perceived as a consumerist idea of sexual rights and the hyperreal notion of ageless sexuality. The specialists seem to anchor their understanding of sexual rights in a biological ground, thereby assigning to 'nature' a boundary-making role.

There are other sites of medical resistance challenging the viagrization of sexuality. In the U.S. the New View Campaign aims to challenge 'the distorted and oversimplified messages about sexuality that pharmaceutical companies use' (New View Campaign 2016). The simplified messages about penile blood flow fail to take into account a broad range of factors influencing older men's sexuality, including psychological factors. There is a strong association between ED and psychological factors such as depression (Araujo et al. 1998; Lexchin 2006). Indeed, research has indicated that what older people think and feel about their sexuality has a more significant influence on sexual desire than biomedical factors (DeLamater & Sill 2005), but these factors are often ignored (Lexchin 2006; Tiefer 1994). Statistics on the prevalence of ED measure physical changes in erectile function rather than emotional responses (Wentzell & Salmerón 2009), and older men may struggle to find comprehensive information or support that explores what erections mean to them and to their partners. Tiefer (1994, p. 373) sums up the problem by noting that:

> Men enter the system innocently looking to understand the cause of a change in their bodily and sexual experience; the options they are given for understanding and coping shape an ever more phallocentric experience. Their partners and any ideas or feelings those partners might have are usually irrelevant to the process. Erections are presented as understandable and manipulable in and of themselves, unhooked from person or script or relationship. A discourse of vascular processes.

Vascular discourses do not take into account the ways that older men experience the changes in the body that occur with age, nor do they take into account the experiences and needs of their partners.

Tipping the balance: women's experiences/ embodied vaginas

The viagrization of older people's sexuality affects older women in a number of ways. Firstly, in the phallocentric focus on older men's sexuality, the experiences and needs of women are dismissed. Women are only present in these discourses in terms of their vaginal needs (Tiefer 1994).

Viagra privileges men's power (Tiefer 1994) and increases the inequality between men and women by giving men more power (Potts et al. 2003). This was highlighted by Potts et al. (2003), who interviewed 27 New Zealand women (aged 33–65 years) whose partners used Viagra. Women reported that Viagra precipitated sudden and unwanted changes in relationships, especially where the women had adjusted to ARED. The women also reported that Viagra changed their partner's communication about sex; there was less negotiation and they felt pressure to engage in sex they did not want. The extent to which women felt empowered to negotiate sexual consent varied considerably. Women in marriages where it was considered their duty to meet their husband's sexual demands were less able to negotiate.

These power imbalances need to be understood in their historical context. In many Western countries, women were expected to meet their husband's sexual needs and men were exempt from criminal liability for raping their wives. Challenges to the marital immunity for rape did not take place until the 1970s and 1980s in many Western countries (Larcombe & Heath 2012), and the United Nations (2015) estimates that more than 42 countries still do not have laws to address this violence. Consequently, many older men have grown up with a sense of sexual entitlement and power. While the legislation has changed in many countries, some older men's behaviour has not. Viagra may be used to advantage in sexual assault (Kintz et al. 2009), and older men may use it to assert what they think are their conjugal rights (Mann et al. 2014).

In addition to an increase in demands for sex, women may experience more subtle forms of sexual pressure when their male partner takes Viagra. Some women believe Viagra will boost male ego and masculinity (Low et al. 2002), and they feel pressure to concede to more frequent sex in order to promote their partner's self-esteem (Potts et al. 2003). Others report pressure to 'make the most of the tablet' and demonstrate a 'normal' and 'healthy' sexuality by matching their partners' enthusiasm for penetrative vaginal sex or risk being labelled 'dysfunctional' themselves (Potts et al. 2003). Women also report that a fear of their partners' infidelity contributes to a sense of pressure to perform sexually (Low et al. 2002; Potts et al. 2003).

The viagrization of older people's sexuality leads to a missed opportunity to build non-penetrative forms of intimacy and sexual activity. Women report being aware of an expectation to demonstrate preference for intercourse over non-coital activities, and while some welcomed a closer relationship, they did not welcome the decrease in time spent on pleasurable activities other than penile-vaginal intercourse (Potts et al. 2003).

In order to resist the viagrization of older people's sexuality, we must look beyond women's vaginal receptivity for penetrative sex – to understanding the embodied desires and needs of older women. For women, sexual arousal and enjoyment are associated with their mental wellbeing (Dunn et al. 1999). The lack of emotional wellbeing and negative emotional feelings during sexual interaction with a partner are more important determinants of sexual distress than impairment of the more physiological aspects of female sexual response (Bancroft et al. 2003).

Some older women enjoy a shift from the passive sexuality of their youth that privileged male pleasure to a sexuality that encompasses a greater variety of non-coital pleasures (Potts et al. 2003). These factors need to be taken into account by older men who want to pleasure their female partners. Women would prefer their male partners discussed Viagra with them before taking it (Low et al. 2002). There is also a need for older men to consider their female partners' emotional needs and to allow time for their partners to adjust emotionally to the physical changes in sexual function that might result from ageing or long intervals between penetrative sex, which might result in painful sex if not taken into account (Kingsberg 2002).

Acknowledging the embodied needs of older women is a key to challenging the viagrization of older people's sexuality and supporting more comprehensive sexual rights for older people. It is also key to resisting medicalised discourses that are emerging related to female sexuality. There has long been a pursuit to match women's libido to men's by developing a female version of Viagra. In 2015 the U.S. Federal Drug Administration (FDA) approved treatment of 'Hypoactive Sexual Desire Disorder' in women (Sprout Pharmaceuticals 2016). The treatment is based on the premise that low sexual desire causes distress and interpersonal difficulty, and a clinical trial has shown significant reductions in distress associated with sexual dysfunction and low sexual desire (Katz et al. 2013). The trial was small, its significance questionable and it did not target older women (it was limited to premenopausal women). However, given the medicalisation of sexuality that occurs across the lifespan, there is a risk that such a treatment will further medicalise older people's sexuality. There is a danger of exacerbating the current genital focus and a failure to understand the importance of comprehensive sexuality education for older people. Such an approach needs to provide information on age-related changes to sexuality for men and women but also outline cultural norms related to sexuality so that older people can critique the current discourses being promoted by pharmaceutical companies.

Sexual norms are cultural not biological

Despite the homogenising global reach of medical understandings of sexuality and ageing, people's ideas of what constitutes 'good' sexuality in older age are diverse. Counter to Western narratives of ageing as decline, slowing or ceasing sexuality over time, ageing is often viewed as a positive bodily change. In India, ageing and attendant decreases in sexual activity can be thought to enhance bodily purity (Lamb 2000). In rural Ghana, older people see decreasing sexual activity as an important way to be a 'respectable' older person, as well as to preserve one's remaining strength after years of hard work (van der Geest 2001). Even in settings where life-long penetrative sex is naturalised as the healthy and ideal form of male sexuality, older people might develop alternative views. For instance, Australian baby boomers reported feeling more 'comfortable in their own skin' as they aged, which led many to feel more free in their sexual self-determination and choices to cease, alter or continue youthful forms of sexuality (Rowntree 2014). Similarly, older Swedish men often came to value non-coital, emotion-laden forms of physical intimacy, rather than to continue penetrative sex or to give up sexual experience (Sandberg 2013; see also Kristiansen & Sandberg in this volume).

This expectation of curtailing sexual activity in older age appears to be ageist and to limit people's right to sexuality from a Western-centric perspective. It assumes all people should have and desire penetrative sex throughout the life course, and that they only stop because of stigma or ill health (e.g. Walz 2002). When looking at these changes in a cultural context, they are in fact the result of people expressing sexual self-determination in settings where ageing bodies themselves are valued. In many cultures, not having sex, either when ritually required or socially appropriate, is highly valued (Sobo & Bell 2001).

Within cultures, people's experiences are not fixed or homogenous. As cultures change, ideas about masculinity, sexuality and whether/how to treat ARED change too. For instance, while the prevalence of decreased erectile function in China has not increased, recent economic and cultural shifts have led men to increase their use of both traditional Chinese and biomedical cures as a way to allay new anxieties related to modernity (Zhang 2015). In addition to cultural change over time, different people within any single society have diverse sexual desires and gender ideals, rooted in variations in psychology, life experience and societal positions in terms of age, class, race and other demographic differences. For example, Portuguese adults experienced similar sexual issues quite differently based on their experiences of gender and the sexual scripts they used, in ways that sometimes conformed to and sometimes challenged dominant medical models of sexuality (Alarcão et al. 2015). Similarly, older people's experiences of ED drug use in New Zealand, where pharmaceuticals are advertised directly to consumers, range widely. Some men happily use ED drugs to perform youthful sexuality and penetration-oriented masculinity into older age, whereas other men and couples report disliking the 'mechanised' feel of pharmaceutically facilitated sex and pre-ferring non-penetrative intimacy (Potts et al. 2004, 2006). Men and women's different socialization often results in different views of sexual issues, as dem-onstrated by research in Japan, which found that both partners in heterosexual couples expected sex to decrease over time, but that women welcomed a shift to more 'sibling-like' relationships, whereas men feared their masculinity would be compromised (Moore 2010).

Considering these cultural and individual differences enables us to think in new ways about the norms for sexuality and masculinity embedded in globalised ED drug marketing and medical practice. Ideas of ageing as decline and of good masculinity as defined by life-long penetrative sex are themselves Western cultural concepts, which may not apply in particular world regions or to people in West-ern cultures who adhere to different ideals of ageing, gender and sexuality. This perspective shows that advocating for older people's sexual rights and sexual self-determination should not be confused with advocating for their ability to access pharmaceuticals to assist with the performance of sexuality cast as 'natural' in West-ern, medical models.

'The Mexican Classic': rejecting ED drugs in Mexico

The experiences of older, working-class Mexican couples demonstrate how cultural context influences people's understandings of sexuality in older age. While men sometimes used sexual interactions with female partners to perform dominance or penetration-oriented masculinities, heterosexual couples also collaborated to reject those aspects of masculinity and sexuality in their responses to decreased erectile function. In urban Mexico, gender norms have been a subject of heated debate for decades. The idea that Mexican men are innately *macho*, or prone to hypersexuality, dominance and emotional closure, is both a common local stereotype and a major topic of societal critique.

Over the course of older Mexican men's lives, ideals of masculinity have shifted from men as financially responsible breadwinners who were expected to engage in frequent extramarital sex to men as emotionally engaged husbands and fathers as well as providers. This context of change influences the ways that older Mexican men and their wives understand men's decreasing erectile function and their expectations for later-life sexuality.

Wentzell's interviews with more than 250 men and heterosexual couples receiving urology treatment in a government-run Cuernavaca, Mexico hospital reveal that despite stereotypes of Mexican men as macho and sex-obsessed, these older, working-class men generally accepted ARED and rejected the idea that it was a medical pathology to be treated with drugs (Wentzell 2013a, 2013b). Instead, many interpreted erectile difficulty as a bodily prompt to abandon their youthful forms of masculinity and embrace what they viewed as a natural shift to an age-appropriate masculinity focused on the domestic sphere and emotional bonds with family. This life course path was so common that one participant called it 'the Mexican classic'; many others described it as embarking on a 'second stage' or 'another plane' of life.

Many older men said that frequent penetrative sex had ceased being important to their definitions of themselves as men. One man explained, 'Erectile dysfunction isn't important. When I was young, it would have been, but not now.' They believed that the decrease in sexual urges they felt as they aged actually enabled them to be better men, in the ways that had become culturally ideal over the courses of their lives. Given this respite from what they saw as macho physical urges, a participant noted 'with age, you start to think more.'

Adopting this understanding was often a collaborative effort, which began when wives told husbands that they understood decrease or cessation of sex in later life as 'natural' and 'normal'. Many men said they initially saw ARED as a failure of manhood, but they came to see it differently with their wives' help. For example, one man said that he had considered seeking medical treatment until his wife said, 'No, better [to let things go] naturally.' She told Wentzell that she welcomed decreasing sex because, 'I've always had less desire.' Similarly, one man said his reduced ability to have penetrative sex made him fear that his wife would cheat. However, she told him that she welcomed this change because, given ageing, menopause and health problems, 'I don't have much desire, I'm not going to look elsewhere.' Both couples reported experiencing increasing emotional closeness as they focused on doing non-sexual activities together. For many couples, this closeness was also enhanced by the fact that men had also stopped or curtailed their extramarital sexual practices. In these cases, rejecting the idea that ARED was a problem to be medicated enabled couples to re-work their relationships in ways that reflected current cultural ideals and that they found mutually satisfying.

The story of the 'Mexican Classic' expectation for sexual change over the life course highlights the influence of cultural contexts on ARED. It provides an opportunity to reflect on the influence of pharmaceutical companies; when men receive messages that ARED is not necessarily pathological, genital changes can be more broadly considered as part of men's and women's whole bodies that are linked to experiences and needs embedded in cultural norms. This case highlights the need to provide older people with comprehensive sexuality education that is culturally sensitive and enables them to question ageist, phallocentric discourses and decide for themselves what they want their sexuality to be.

As anthropologist Gayle Rubin famously noted, sex is like food in that eating is a biological human imperative, but what counts as food varies remarkably across cultures. Similarly, what counts as 'good' sex – or even as sex at all – depends on cultural context (Rubin 1975). Norms regarding manhood are similarly variable, but the globalization of Western assumptions about manliness and male sexuality via ED drug marketing can obscure that reality. Variation in men's ideals and experiences of sexuality across cultures challenges the assumption that penetrative sex throughout the life course is biologically natural and universally socially ideal.

Comprehensive sexuality education as resistance

The concepts of healthy ageing and sexuality need to be broadened to avoid medicalisation and phallocentrism (Tiefer 1996; Potts 2000; Katz & Marshall 2003). Older people's sexual rights would be better ensured through access to comprehensive sexuality education that critiques the viagrization of sexuality and emphasises their right to sexual self-determination in whatever forms that takes. This approach could help those older men who have not thought beyond the coital imperative to think more broadly and to explore what sexuality means to them and to their partners. It could assist them in understanding how sexuality is influenced by culture and encourage them to think critically about which cultural norms they wish to adopt.

This education could include information on:

- The ways in which sexuality is socially constructed and influenced by ageism;
- How penile erections change with age, disease and social experience;
- The importance of men understanding what penile erections mean to them and their sense of masculinity;
- How to initiate conversation with a partner or health practitioner about what it means to be a man and what part sexuality plays in this;
- How to have a conversation with sexual partners about what gives pleasure;
- The importance of intimacy and a broad range of sexual activities (other than penetrative vaginal sex) in creating sexual intimacy and pleasure, supported with explicit information regarding how to have diverse forms of intimacy and pleasure;
- How to discuss libido, including the level of sexual desire and desired frequency of sex, with a sexual partner;
- Negotiating libido mismatch, including fears about infidelity;
- Negotiating sexual consent and reaching agreement about when and how often Viagra is taken and partners have penetrative vaginal or other sex; and
- The importance of allowing time to adjust to changes that ageing and Viagra use can bring to a relationship.

Education could be provided through a range of contacts, including medical practitioners who prescribe Viagra. However, as Tiefer (1994) notes, men seeking to make sense of their ARED face a clinical focus on the hardness and duration of their erections that does not account for men's sexual relationships or knowledge of sexual techniques. Others have suggested that older men may not raise the topic with their general practitioners (and even seek out drugs online to avoid this conversation) because they do not feel they have permission to do so (Gott & Hinchliff 2003; Gott, Hinchliff & Galena 2004; Andrews & Piterman 2007). Doctors could potentially address this problem by initiating conversations about ARED with older patients. It is also important to include older women in this education (Loe 2004b).

Furthermore, while medical interactions have become the default settings for discussing age-related sexual changes in many societies, limiting discussion of this issue to that realm reinforces the medicalisation of sexuality. If other sites that serve older people – from private activity clubs, to continuing education programs, to senior living and care facilities – host discussions of these issues, the messages will spread more broadly and people will feel more able to adopt diverse rather than medically normative sexual practices.

Conclusion

In this chapter we have argued that a rights-based approach to older people's sexuality cannot simply result in a view that older men taking Viagra are asserting their right to enjoy the benefits of scientific progress. Rather, we proposed that a sexual rights lens requires a more comprehensive, less phallocentric approach that takes into account the perspectives of female partners and the cultural norms in which older people are situated. Older people have the right to information that enables them to critique ageist norms that emphasise penetrative sex. To achieve this level of empowerment, comprehensive sexuality education needs to be provided to older people in such a way that the messages of choice informed by critical thought ring louder than the message that Viagra is the solution to every problem. Until we do this, pharmaceutical companies will continue to dominate and thus shape cultural norms about sexuality and ageing.

References

Alarcão, V., Fernando, L. and Giami, A., 2015. Traditions and contradictions of sexual function definitions for Portuguese heterosexual men and women: Medicalization and socially constructed gender effects. *Sexual and Relationship Therapy, 31*(3), pp. 1–18.

Andrews, C.N. and Piterman, L., 2007. Sex and the older man: GP perceptions and management. *Australian Family Physician, 36*(10), p. 867.

Araujo, A.B., Durante, R., Feldman, H.A., Goldstein, I. and McKinlay, J.B., 1998. The relationship between depressive symptoms and male erectile dysfunction: Cross-sectional results from the Massachusetts male aging study. *Psychosomatic Medicine, 60*(4), pp. 458–465.

Associated Press, 2013. Pfizer to sell viagra online, in first for big pharma: AP. *CBS news online.* www.cbsnews.com/news/pfizer-to-sell-viagra-online-in-first-for-big-pharma-ap/

Baglia, J., 2005. *The Viagra ad venture: Masculinity, marketing, and the performance of sexual health,* Peter Lang, New York.

Bancroft, J., Loftus, J. and Long, J.S., 2003. Distress about sex: A national survey of women in heterosexual relationships. *Archives of Sexual Behavior, 32*(3), pp. 193–208.

Calasanti, T. and King, N., 2005. Firming the floppy penis: Age, class, and gender relations in the lives of old men. *Men and Masculinities, 8*(1), pp. 3–23.

Caplan, A. and Elliott, C., 2004. Is it ethical to use enhancement technologies to make us better than well? *PLoS Med, 1*(3), p. e52.

Connell, R.W. and Messerschmidt, J.W., 2005. Hegemonic masculinity rethinking the concept. *Gender & Society, 19*(6), pp. 829–859.

Conrad, P. and Leiter, V., 2004. Medicalization, markets and consumers. *Journal of Health and Social Behavior, 45*, pp. 158–176.

DeLamater, J. D., & Sill, M. 2005. Sexual desire in later life. *Journal of Sex Research, 42*(2), pp. 138–149.

Dunn, K.M., Croft, P.R. and Hackett, G.I., 1999. Association of sexual problems with social, psychological, and physical problems in men and women: A cross sectional population survey. *Journal of Epidemiology and Community Health, 53*(3), pp. 144–148.

Ferrero Camoletto, R. and Bertone, C., 2017. Medicalized virilism under scrutiny: Expert knowledge on male sexual health in Italy. In A. King, A.C. Santos, I. Crowhurst (eds.), *Sexuality in theory and practice: Insights and critical debates from Europe and beyond.* Routledge, London, vol. 7, pp. 196–209.

Ferrero Camoletto, R., Bertone, C. and Salis, F., 2015. Medicalizing male underperformance: Expert discourses on male sexual health in Italy. *Salute e Società*, 1EN, pp. 183–205

Gott, M., 2004. *Sexuality, sexual health and ageing*, Open University Press/McGraw-Hill Education, Maidenhead, UK.

Gott, M., 2006. Sexual health and the new ageing. *Age and Ageing, 35*(2), pp. 106–107.

Gott, M. and Hinchliff, S., 2003. How important is sex in later life? The views of older people. *Social Science & Medicine, 56*(8), pp. 1617–1628.

Gott, M., Hinchliff, S. and Galena, E., 2004. General practitioner attitudes to discussing sexual health issues with older people. *Social Science & Medicine, 58*(11), pp. 2093–2103.

Gross, G., and Blundo, R. 2005. Viagara: Medical technology constructing aging masculinity. *Journal of Sociology & Social Welfare, 32*, pp. 85–97.

Jones, J. and Pugh, S., 2005. Ageing gay men: Lessons from the sociology of embodiment. *Men and Masculinities, 7*(3), pp. 248–260.

Katz, M., DeRogatis, L.R., Ackerman, R., Hedges, P., Lesko, L., Garcia, M. and Sand, M., 2013. Efficacy of flibanserin in women with hypoactive sexual desire disorder: Results from the BEGONIA trial. *The Journal of Sexual Medicine, 10*(7), pp. 1807–1815.

Katz, S., 2001. Growing older without aging? Positive aging, anti-ageism, and anti-aging. *Generations, 25*(4), p. 27.

Katz, S. and Marshall, B., 2003. New sex for old: Lifestyle, consumerism, and the ethics of aging well. *Journal of Aging Studies, 17*(1), pp. 3–16.

Kingsberg, S.A., 2002. The impact of aging on sexual function in women and their partners. *Archives of Sexual Behavior, 31*(5), pp. 431–437.

Kintz, P., Evans, J., Villain, M., Chatterton, C. and Cirimele, V., 2009. Hair analysis to demonstrate administration of sildenafil to a woman in a case of drug-facilitated sexual assault. *Journal of Analytical Toxicology, 33*(8), pp. 553–556.

Lamb, S., 2000. *White saris and sweet mangoes: Aging, gender, and body in North India*, University of California Press, Berkeley, CA.

Lamb, S., 2014. Permanent personhood or meaningful decline? Toward a critical anthropology of successful aging. *Journal of Aging Studies, 29*, pp. 41–52.

Lamb, S., 2015. Beyond the view of the west: Ageing and anthropology. In J. Twigg and W. Martin (eds.), *Handbook of cultural gerontology*. Routledge, London and New York.

Lamb, S. (ed.), 2017. *Successful aging? Global perspectives on a contemporary obsession*, Rutgers University Press, New Brunswick, NJ.

Larcombe, W. and Heath, M., 2012. Developing the common law and rewriting the history of rape in marriage in Australia: PGA v The Queen. *Sydney Law Review, 34*, p. 785.

Lexchin, J., 2006. Bigger and better: How Pfizer redefined erectile dysfunction. *PLoS Med, 3*(4), p. e132.

Lodge, A.C. and Umberson, D., 2013. Age and embodied masculinities: Midlife gay and heterosexual men talk about their bodies. *Journal of Aging Studies, 27*(3), pp. 225–232.

Loe, M., 2001. Fixing broken masculinity: Viagra as a technology for the production of gender and sexuality. *Sexuality and Culture, 5*(3), pp. 97–125.

Loe, M., 2004a. *The rise of Viagra: How the little blue pill changed sex in America*, NYU Press, New York.

Loe, M., 2004b. Sex and the senior woman: Pleasure and danger in the viagra era. *Sexualities, 7*(3), pp. 303–326.

Low, W.Y., Zulkifli, S.N., Wong, Y.L. and Tan, H.M., 2002. What Malaysian women believe about viagra: A qualitative inquiry. *The Aging Male, 5*(1), pp. 57–63.

Mann, R., Horsley, P., Barrett, C. and Tinney, J., 2014. *Norma's project: A research study into the sexual assault of older women in Australia* (ARCSHS Monograph Series No. 98), Melbourne: Australian Research Centre in Sex, Health and Society, La Trobe University.

Marshall, B.L., 2010. Science, medicine and virility surveillance: 'Sexy seniors' in the pharmaceutical imagination. *Sociology of Health & Illness, 32*(2), pp. 211–224.

Marshall, B.L., 2011. The graying of 'sexual health': A critical research agenda. *Canadian Review of Sociology/Revue canadienne de sociologie, 48*(4), pp. 390–413.

Marshall, B.L., 2012. Medicalization and the refashioning of age-related limits on sexuality. *Journal of Sex Research, 49*(4), pp. 337–343.

Moore, K.L., 2010. Sexuality and sense of self in later life: Japanese men's and women's reflections on sex and aging. *Journal of Cross-Cultural Gerontology, 25*(2), pp. 149–163.

New View Campaign, 2016, Challenging the medicalization of sex, viewed March 2016 www.newviewcampaign.org/default.asp

Pantalone, D. W., Bimbi, D. S., and Parsons, J. T. 2008. Motivations for the recreational use of erectile enhancing medications in urban gay and bisexual men. *Sexually Transmitted Infections, 84*(6), pp. 458–462.

Pfizer, 2016, Learning: What is ED? Pfizer, viewed March 2016 www.viagra.com/learning/what-is-ed

Potts, A., 2000. 'The essence of the hard on' hegemonic masculinity and the cultural construction of 'Erectile Dysfunction'. *Men and Masculinities, 3*(1), pp. 85–103.

Potts, A., Gavey, N., Grace, V.M. and Vares, T., 2003. The downside of viagra: Women's experiences and concerns. *Sociology of Health & Illness, 25*(7), pp. 697–719.

Potts, A., Grace, V.M., Gavey, N. and Vares, T., 2004. 'Viagra stories': Challenging 'erectile dysfunction'. *Social Science & Medicine, 59*(3), pp. 489–499.

Potts, A., Grace, V.M., Vares, T. and Gavey, N., 2006. 'Sex for life'? Men's counter-stories on 'erectile dysfunction', male sexuality and ageing. *Sociology of Health & Illness, 28*(3), pp. 306–329.

Riska, E., 2003. Gendering the medicalization thesis. In M. S. Segal and V. Demos (eds.), *Gender perspectives on health and healing: Key themes: Advances in gender research*. Vol. 7. Oxford, Elsevier, pp. 59–87.

Rowntree, M.R., 2014. 'Comfortable in my own skin': A new form of sexual freedom for ageing baby boomers. *Journal of Aging Studies*, vol. 31, pp. 150–158.

Rubin, G., 1975. The traffic in women. In R. Reiter (ed.), *Toward an anthropology of women*. Monthly Review Press, New York., pp. 157–210.

Sandberg, L., 2013. Just feeling a naked body close to you: Men, sexuality and intimacy in later life. *Sexualities*, *16*(3–4), pp. 261–282.

Slevin, K.F. and Linneman, T.J., 2010. Old gay men's bodies and masculinities. *Men and Masculinities*, *12*(4), pp. 483–507.

Sobo, E.J., and Bell, S., 2001. Celibacy in cross-cultural perspective: An overview. In E. J. Sobo and S. Bell (eds.), *Celibacy, culture and society: The anthropology of sexual abstinence*. The University of Wisconsin Press, Madison, pp. 3–26.

Sprout Pharmaceuticals, 2016, Meet Addyi: The first of her kind, viewed March 2016, www.addyi.com/

Tiefer, L., 1986. In pursuit of the perfect penis: The medicalization of male sexuality. *American Behavioral Scientist*, *29*(5), pp. 579–599.

Tiefer, L., 1994. The medicalization of impotence: Normalizing phallocentrism. *Gender & Society*, *8*(3), pp. 363–377.

Tiefer, L., 1996. The medicalization of sexuality: Conceptual, normative, and professional issues. *Annual Review of Sex Research*, *7*(1), pp. 252–282.

United Nations, 2015. Progress of the world's women 2015–2016. Transforming economies, realising rights. United Nations. http://progress.unwomen.org/en/2015/download/

Van der Geest, S., 2001. 'No strength': Sex and old age in a rural town in Ghana. *Social Science & Medicine*, *53*(10), pp. 1383–1396.

Walz, T., 2002. Crones, dirty old men, sexy seniors: Representations of the sexuality of older persons. *Journal of Aging and Identity*, *7*(2), pp. 99–112.

Wentzell, E., 2011. Marketing silence, public health stigma and the discourse of risky gay viagra use in the US. *Body & Society*, *17*(4), pp. 105–125.

Wentzell, E.A., 2013a. Aging respectably by rejecting medicalization: Mexican men's reasons for not using erectile dysfunction drugs. *Medical Anthropology Quarterly*, *27*(1), pp. 3–22.

Wentzell, E.A., 2013b. *Maturing masculinities: Aging, chronic illness, and viagra in Mexico*, Duke University Press, Durham, NC.

Wentzell, E. and Salmerón, J., 2009. Prevalence of erectile dysfunction and its treatment in a Mexican population: Distinguishing between erectile function change and dysfunction. *Journal of Men's Health*, *6*(1), pp. 56–62.

Zhang, Y.Z., 2015. *Impotence epidemic*, Duke University Press, Durham, NC.

11

OLDER PEOPLE AS CYBER-SEXUAL BEINGS

Online and internet dating

Sue Malta and Summer Roberts

Online dating appears to be a global phenomenon and is now firmly established in industrialised countries around the world as a socially acceptable means to find new partners (Finkel et al. 2012). A recent worldwide study of 25,200 people (12,600 cohabiting couples), for instance, found that one-third had used online dating websites and 15% of these were in a relationship that began online (Hogan et al. 2011).

Older people are disproportionately more likely than those who are younger to use online dating as a way to find their current partner (Hogan et al. 2011). In addition, older adults aged 55+ are reportedly the fastest growing segment on dating websites (Experian Hitwise 2012; Fairfax Digital 2012). Although academic evidence supporting this claim is difficult to find, the recent proliferation of niche dating sites catering specifically to older people, such as Senior Friend Finder®, Singles Over 60®, and Our Time®, indicates the market is responding to increases in consumer demand. Furthermore, evidence suggests that older people represent the fastest developing sector of Internet users (Australian Bureau of Statistics [ABS] 2011; Perrin & Duggan 2015). In the US, for instance, older people's usage of the Internet jumped from 14% in 2000 to 58% in 2015 (Perrin & Duggan 2015). In Australia the figures are similar, with 10% of older people using the Internet in 2001 (ABS 2003), compared to 68% in 2013–2014 (Australian Communications & Media Authority 2015).

Single older people appreciate and desire dating and sexual relationships (Malta & Farquharson 2014). In national samples of older adults aged 57–85 in the US, for example, 14% report being in dating relationships (Brown & Shinohara 2013). Similarly in Australia, online dating membership rates for older people indicate that large numbers are either dating or looking for a dating partner (Fairfax Digital 2012, 2010; Fairfax Media 2010). Dating, particularly online dating, offers the opportunity to explore alternatives for new partnerships, although heterosexual women and men can demonstrate different initial goals for companionship and intimacy (McWilliams & Barrett 2014). Older women generally date for companionship while maintaining independence rather than in hopes of marriage, whereas men more commonly report seeking marital partners in later life (McWilliams & Barrett 2014; Watson & Stelle 2011). Yet, both heterosexual women and men look for relationships that are romantic and sexually intimate (Malta & Farquharson 2014). Similarly, gay men and lesbians across age groups – those who live in European countries accepting of same-sex relationships and the opportunity for same-sex marriage – tend to express greater desire for long-term relationships and monogamy through their online dating profiles (Potârcă, Mills & Neberich 2015). Furthermore, a recent study conducted by Match.com surveyed a nationally representative sample of LGBTQ people aged 18–70+ who used online dating websites and found that more than 53% hoped to eventually marry (PR Newswire 2016).

This chapter examines the new frontier of online dating and the potential it offers older people in terms of the increased possibility of identifying a suitable partner and making dating easier. We also explore the sexual rights of older people in light of opportunities and limitations presented by the internet. We then consider the implications for policy and practice of online dating sites providing ageing members with the necessary protections and information for maintaining their sexual health and wellbeing.

Increasing partner selection, choices and information

Although some older people may no longer be sexually active, this choice usually reflects social and psychological reasons rather than any physical or biological imperative (Hillman 2000; Zeiss & Kasl-Godley 2001). Some studies have shown that interest in sexual activity wanes with age (Waite et al. 2009), but others have found ongoing sexual interest even in the very-old (Beckman et al. 2008; Lindau et al. 2007). Waning sexual interest among women, some as young as 50 years of age, commonly results from a lack of available sexual partners. For instance, older women are more likely than older men to be un-partnered, mostly due to demographic ageing factors, but also as a result of the intersection of ageism and sexism limiting their opportunities (Carpenter, Nathanson & Kim 2006). Older lesbians also appear to experience lessening of sexual activity around age 55, but this change accompanies a qualitative shift for some from sexual intimacy in favour of a focus on emotional closeness (Averett, Yoon & Jenkins 2012). Likewise, older gay men appear to experience a lessening of sexual activity compared to their younger counterparts and are less likely to have casual sex partners with increasing age (Lyons et al. 2010). Ill health and disability in later life can also affect sexual desire and/ or activity for both men and women, particularly when one applies sexual intercourse – penile-vaginal penetration – as the 'gold standard' by which sexual activity is judged (Hinchliff & Gott 2004).

Despite these challenges, many older people embrace their health limitations and learn to adapt by becoming more sexually creative, and they report being more sexually fulfilled as a result (DeLamater 2012; Hurd Clarke 2006; Malta 2013). Ongoing sexual expression is also associated with lower levels of depression (Ganong & Larson 2011), increased self-esteem (Kontual & Haavio-Mannila 2009), health and wellbeing (Anderson 2013; Bach et al. 2014; Woloski-Wruble et al. 2010), as well as overall quality of life (Rosen & Bachmann 2008).

Access to the Internet and online dating provides older people with the tools to explore and enhance their sexual expression, by providing the possibility of engaging in erotica, pornography and cybersex (Adams, Oye & Parker 2003; Malta 2007). Likewise, the Internet provides access to sex information (Berdychevsky & Nimrod 2015; Daneback et al. 2012), at a time in older people's lives when such information is not generally forthcoming from their personal physicians due to embedded ageist beliefs regarding late life asexuality (Hinchliff 2015). Under such circumstances the Internet becomes the 'preferred source' for information about sexual health matters as it helps to circumvent 'potentially awkward discussions' (Scaunich 2014). As Adams and colleagues state:

> The Internet allows older adults to socialize despite limitations with mobility and physical impairments. It also allows them to educate themselves about changes they may experience in their sexuality and to explore and experiment with the more intimate aspects of themselves anonymously, affordably, and immediately. This is not only true for seniors living in North America, but globally.
>
> *(Adams et al. 2003: 413)*

Online dating and the Internet can thus provide older people with the freedom and the means to explore and experience themselves as sexual/cyber-sexual beings, at a time when society denies them this right. For instance, even when Canadian newspaper and magazine articles highlight older people's interest in and experiences with sexual activity, authors of these articles still demonstrate an ageist bias in their writing by focusing on diminishing sexual interests and functioning, as well as medicalising and emphasising sexual decline (Wada, Clarke & Rozanova 2015).

Historically, this ageist bias extended to sexuality research. Many large-scale national studies specifically excluded respondents over the age of 60, such as the first wave of the Australian Study of Health and Relationships (ASHR: Minichiello, Plummer & Macklin 2003; Richters & Rissel 2005) and similar studies in the UK (Johnson et al. 2001) and the US (Laumann, Paik & Rosen 1999). This bias also extended to early explorations of older people's online sexual and dating behaviours, with very few studies undertaken with samples aged 60 and older (see Döring 2009 for discussion).

Recently, however, the late-life sexual landscape has changed. There has been a groundswell of interest in this area, and more contemporary studies have sought to include adults 60 years and older for the first time, such as the National Social Life, Health, and Aging Project (US: Lindau et al. 2007), the most recent National Survey of Sexual Attitudes and Lifestyles (UK), the second wave of the ASHR study

(Australia), and the Global Study of Sexual Attitudes and Behaviors (Laumann et al. 2006; Nicolosi et al. 2004). Much of the research on older people's sexual behaviour, welcome though it is, is almost always narrowly defined, as it primarily focuses on middle-class heterosexuals (DeLamater 2012). Older LGBTI people are noticeably absent from many sexuality studies, as are racial or ethnic minorities (Novak 2016).

Providing structure to the dating 'game'

Older people enjoy using dating websites to search for and find new romantic and intimate relationships (Malta & Farquharson 2014). Dating websites offer a structured approach to dating that can provide a relief for the newly single emerging from long-term marriages (Malta 2013) and re-entering the 'dating game' (Jönson & Siverskog 2012). Furthermore, online dating also provides a welcome alternative to the bar and club scene (Whitty & Carr 2006), which many older people find uncomfortable or dissatisfying (McWilliams & Barrett 2014; Stephure et al. 2009). In addition, online dating offers older people a much larger pool of potential partners compared to the limited number available in their offline networks (Illouz 2007; Rosenfeld & Thomas 2012). It also allows a number of relationships to be considered before a commitment is made and lessens the need to persevere with a relationship that is not 'quite right' (Malta & Farquharson 2014). Moreover, online dating changes the way older people experience new relationships: it breaks down barriers to communication and allows those who are less socially confident to become more so. Online dating also redefines social rules and conventions, as many older heterosexual women act as initiators in their new relationships by making the first contact, rather than waiting for men to make the first move (Malta 2013).

The goal of most relationships initiated through dating websites is to meet in real life, regardless of whether the intention is for pursuing casual versus permanent or predominantly sexual relationships (Couch & Liamputtong 2008; Whitty & Carr 2006). For older people, the process of searching for and initiating new relationships through dating websites and moving them offline can be exciting and stimulating, both mentally and physically/sexually, particularly as the relationships usually become sexually intimate within a few weeks of meeting face to face (Malta & Farquharson 2014). For many older people, finding new partners in late life and enjoying new sexual outlets appears to be both a fulfiling and liberating experience.

The challenges

The Internet offers older people choices and opportunities to express their sexuality, but it also presents a number of challenges that have not been well recognised. In the following section we outline the challenges, including misrepresentation and deception, ageism and the lack of information on safer sexual practices.

Misrepresentation and deception

Online dating websites emerge as a particularly valuable method for older people seeking new relationships due to the difficulties they face in their offline networks for finding romantic and sexual partners (Rosenfeld & Thomas 2012). However, these websites also present potential challenges in the form of misrepresentation and deception. Although misrepresentation and deception are common concerns among those who use the Internet (Hall et al. 2010), deception is limited to a minority of users (Caspi & Gorsky 2006). Within online dating websites, misrepresentation tends to be tied to constructing an attractive profile and is relatively minor in scale, including more common misrepresentations made by men regarding their education and income, women regarding their weight, and older people about their age (Hall et al. 2010; Toma, Hancock & Ellison 2008). Perhaps more harmful, online scams – including romance scams occurring through online dating – have become relatively well-known and carry potentially great psychological and monetary consequences for victims (Buchanan & Whitty 2014; Cross, Smith & Richards 2014; Rege 2009; Whitty & Buchanan 2012).

Researchers have postulated that older people may be especially vulnerable to online romance scams (Cross, Smith & Richards 2014). However, a recent Australian study found this was more likely the case for adults aged 40–54 (Jorna 2016). Predatory behaviours, including cyberstalking (McFarlane & Bocij 2003; Pittaro 2007) and dating violence following online meetings (Cali, Coleman & Campbell 2013), pose potential dangers that contribute to both individual and institutional concerns surrounding online dating. Other research comparing university students to housing authority residents (the majority of whom were over 50 years of age) found that older people, especially older women, lacked an understanding of Internet security needs (Grimes et al. 2010). This is reinforced by more recent research, which shows that those aged 65 and older are more likely to be victims of what is termed 'computer support fraud', perpetrated by people masquerading as representatives of so-called legitimate companies, who offer to fix problems with recipients' computers (Jorna 2016).

Ageism online

Online dating provides greater opportunities for older people than traditional means of meeting partners, but the online environment also has the potential for reinforcing ageism in the dating world and beyond. For instance, the dating profiles of some older LGBTI people incorporate self-deprecating jokes about their ageing in an attempt to construct a self-presentation that combines a sense of humour and honesty. However, by advertising that they are still 'interested in sex, *despite* their age' and by 'praising youthfulness' and asking that age be 'viewed as irrelevant', they unintentionally reproduce the idea of old age as problematic (Jönson & Siverskog 2012). Jagger (2005) also found that older men and women used qualifying statements such as "young 55" or "fun loving very fit 50+" to distance themselves from their chronological age.

In addition, a quantitative study of 4,000 US online dating profiles showed that older people's descriptions contained more references to health and money, perhaps reflecting attempts to avoid stereotypical issues associated with ageing such as loss, inadequacy and dependence (Davis & Fingerman 2016). A similar quantitative analysis of 200 online dating profiles comparing heterosexual individuals aged 65 and older to those between 25 and 35 found that the older daters tended to be more selective than younger daters when identifying what they wanted in a partner, including expressing a desire for younger partners (McIntosh et al. 2011).

In qualitative research with adults aged 50-plus, analysis of participants' accounts of their online dating experiences and their online profiles also highlighted a preference for younger partners, as well as attempts to present the self as youthful (McWilliams & Barrett 2014). Older women especially note the ageist lens through which others view their sexuality (Rowntree 2014) and how age and gender biases – the double standard of ageism and sexism (Sontag 1972) – are obstacles that must be overcome in online dating as well as in their offline lives (Fileborn et al. 2015).

Sexually Transmissible Infections (STIs)

The lack of sex education prior to the 1960s and an absence of contemporary safe-sex campaigns targeting older people (Sherrard & Wainwright 2013) may have impacted – and is likely to continue to impact for some time – older people's ongoing sexual expression and/or their realisation of the need to practice safe sex (Nash et al. 2015). Greater understanding of the sexual health needs of older people is imperative, especially given evidence showing that rates of STIs and, to a lesser extent, HIV/AIDS among older people are steadily increasing around the world (Minichiello, Hawkes & Pitts 2011). Additionally, in the US, only a minority of older adults report regularly using condoms or being tested for STIs (Schick et al. 2010).

A number of studies in younger populations showed the Internet may potentially act as a pathway in the likelihood of contracting an STI, due to the increased number of offline sexual meetings possible (see Couch & Liamputtong 2008 for discussion). More current research on sexual practices among individuals meeting romantic partners online demonstrates conflicting results. Compared to meeting sexual partners in person, online daters do not necessarily consider their risks of contracting STIs as higher (Couch, Liamputtong & Pitts 2012). However, women who have sex with individuals they meet online do tend to use condoms and get tested for STIs more frequently (McFarlane et al. 2004). Older women particularly are more likely than younger women to broach the topic of STIs with sexual partners they meet online, but they are also less likely to refuse having sex with a partner they met online who does not want to use a condom (Bateson et al. 2012).

The sheer accessibility of a myriad of sexual partners through online dating may increase the exposure of older people to STIs, particularly given the growing numbers who find new partners through such a medium (Bateson et al. 2012), as well as the level of sexual risk taking amongst older people (Amin 2016). Although such risks have yet to be determined, such a possibility raises concerns about older people's rights to access comprehensive, non-ageist and sex-positive sexuality education. Many online dating services promote safe-sex messages as well as the safe use of their websites, but with very few exceptions, they mostly ignore older people. Orel and colleagues found there was very little information available offline either, and the little that was obtainable did not meet acceptable criteria for older adult use (Orel, Spence & Steele 2005; Orel, Wright & Wagner 2004). The results are concerning and a reflection of the ageist presumption regarding late-life asexuality. This ageist bias also appears to extend to sexual rights and the Internet.

Sexual rights and the Internet: where do older people fit in?

Growing recognition is given to the valuable role that the Internet plays in advancing sexual rights (Global Information Society Watch [GISWatch] 2015: 5) and further, that 'internet rights' are now seen as 'human rights' (Association of Progressive Communications 2015). GISWatch calls for:

> . . . understanding of how the internet can ensure that muted voices are heard, that connections can be made with relative safety thanks to the capacity to determine the lines between what is private and what is public online, and that the internet still provides an open space for imagining and constructing alternative ways of relating, living and being.
>
> *(GISWatch 2015: 5–6)*

The Internet is now seen as a legitimate forum for sexual expression, exploration of sexual identity and source of sex education (GISWatch 2015). Although these major advances are laudable, many of the concerns of the Internet rights organisations that champion this space focus on young people, women and developing countries. Older people as a population group appear to be missing from their purview and, as such, lack a legitimate body advocating for them. So, although online dating presents new opportunities for older people to explore their sexuality, the medium also poses potential issues with regard to their sexual rights.

As mentioned earlier in this book, the World Health Organisation's (WHO) charter on *Sexual health, human rights and the law* (WHO 2015) provides information and protection in this respect. First, older people must be able to seek sexual and romantic partners free from discrimination, restriction or degradation tied to their sexual orientation, gender identity, ethnicity or disability (see Sexual Rights 1, 2 and 4). Although these rights apply across the life span, they play a role in limiting older people's access to online dating. In early 2015, media outlets highlighted the ageist practice of Tinder Plus, an app for online dating that charges users in the US and UK up to twice as much for upgraded services if they are at least 30 years of age (see, for example, Bisceglio 2015; Sanders 2015). Similarly, gay men and lesbians have faced exclusion from particular online dating sites, specifically eHarmony. Following court battles, the website created a site specifically for gay and lesbian singles and eventually merged it with eHarmony (DeFalco 2008; eHarmony 2009, 2010), but this example highlights how practices in the online dating industry can infringe older people's sexual rights.

Second, older people must be able to begin sexual relationships by their own choice and without fear of sexual violence and coercion (see Sexual Rights 3, 5, 6 and 11). These rights indicate that older people engaging in online dating should have the freedom and autonomy to seek new relationships online, to have the choice to veto unsuitable partners and to participate in sexual experiences, as desired, and to do so safely and securely in environments that provide security and protection of personal information online or offline. Although typical online dating websites provide precautions and safety guidelines to users planning to meet others online, blanket warnings may be easily overlooked. Following a 2011 lawsuit against Match.com by a woman who was sexually assaulted on a date, the online dating website began screening its members (Stone 2011), a practice eHarmony claimed to already have in place (CNN Wire Staff 2011). However, neither site reported conducting full background checks of its members (eHarmony.com 2016; Match.com 2016). Instead, these sites, as well as others, rely on blog postings and advice columns on separate webpages to provide users with steps to follow for protecting their safety. Older people may not be aware of this important information.

If members so choose, they can opt to pay outside services to run background checks on their potential dates (Rosenbloom 2010). And some states in the US, including Illinois, New Jersey, New York and Texas, have passed legislation designed to protect their citizens who participate in online dating by requiring sites to report whether they screen members. As yet, however, no federal legislation exists, and how much these laws actually protect online daters remains questionable (Horcher 2012; Jayson 2014). These loopholes contribute to older people's vulnerability to sexual violence and coercion and need to be addressed.

Third, older people must be able to access information and education on sexuality and sexual health, including resources promoting sex positivity that are both age appropriate and easily accessible, in order to enjoy and maintain the highest possible level of health, pleasure, sexuality and wellbeing (see Sexual Rights 7, 8, 9 and 10). Although the Internet contains vast amounts of information on health and sexuality, guidance on what literature is valid and how to locate it is typically not linked from online dating sites. As has been shown to be the case with printed materials, much of the information is skewed towards a much younger population (Orel, Wright & Wagner 2004), again, due to the ageist assumption that older people are not sexually active and therefore won't require sexual health education. A Google search with the search terms "sexual health after 60" turns up a plethora of information aimed at an older demographic, but the legitimacy (or accuracy) of the available information is questionable. For instance, one such search produced over nine million results, but the first page provided nothing but links to advice sites boasting how to have "hot" sex after 60, and references to so-called 'medical' information was limited to websites such as WebMD and the Mayo Clinic. Furthermore, whereas online websites that encourage maintaining an active sex life might appear to provide an alternative to ageist stereotypes, they likely do little to educate older people about how to avoid STIs by engaging in safer sex practices.

Regardless of these factors, which need to be addressed, the impact of the Internet and online dating is generally positive, providing opportunities for connection that might not otherwise be possible and changing the way older people experience their new relationships and themselves.

Implications for policy and practice

Across the world, people may be uninformed about what constitutes the 'normative patterns of ageing' and, subsequently, they may resort to stereotypes as a way to make sense of sexuality amongst older people (Burgess 2004: 439). Although older people have remained for many years in our collective conscious as being asexual, the current groundswell in public and research interest in late-life sexuality is redefining the perception of asexuality to 'sexy oldie' (see Chapter 1). Despite this perceptual shift in community attitudes, ageing sexuality continues to be invisible at the policy level. For instance, in government-mandated health care policies around the world, the sexual health needs of older people are often completely omitted or mentioned only cursorily. A recent scoping review of Australian and international federal policy documents reinforced this argument. In Australia, for instance, it found no evidence of 'any policy specific to midlife and older adult sexuality and sexual health' (Kirkman, Kenny & Fox 2013: 137), a situation reflected in both the US (Centers for Disease Control 2011) and the UK (Gott 2005) and globally (World Health Organisation 2015).

Despite this lack of representation at the state and federal government level, smaller grassroots organisations such as the Australian Women's Health in the South-East (WHISE) and the US Woodhall Sexual Freedom Alliance (WSFA) have recognised the need to address the deficits in this area.

Recommendations for the future

Online dating sites can provide older people with initial exposure to new romantic and sexual relations; these sites are therefore uniquely poised to offer guidance specifically on sexual health and sex positivity more generally. The challenges presented by online dating also provide key factors for action.

Regarding online misrepresentation and deception, rather than having safety tips filed away under "Help" or on a separate page with more general dating advice, the information should be presented to consumers before they begin to construct their personal profiles – perhaps in a section entitled "important concerns for those new to online dating". Paid online dating sites could also consider collecting more specific forms of identification from new users (such as driver's licence information).

Such a requirement could enable automatic entry of information in dating profiles, including age, and would confirm that the person who created the profile was actually the person in the profile. Integration of optional background checks into the services offered by these sites or requiring criminal background checks of all members might also be worthwhile, in order to provide members with assurance that other users are not engaging in scams.

Structural changes are necessary to help combat ageist stereotypes online. For instance, dating websites have the potential to contribute to a declining emphasis on age in the way they develop and market their services. By providing age ranges rather than members' specific chronological age, or even removing age as a central characteristic in personal profiles, this would allow users to share their age if and when desired, and may help discourage ageism among online daters. Likewise, limiting the use of advertisements and commercials presenting unattainable images of ageing and presenting more realistic images of older people could also alleviate older members feeling as if they must measure up to a certain standard.

Regarding inaccessible and limited information on STIs, online dating websites could incorporate specific guidance by public health professionals on the use of male and female condoms. This guidance could also direct members where to go for reliable sexual health information as well as provide links to community health services, to provide older people with the sexual health resources they need to empower themselves as sexual beings.

Without appropriate recognition of the dating and sexual behaviours of this population by governments, the medical field and other service providers, suitable health and education programs cannot be designed to ensure sex-positive messages are reaching older people. Failure to recognise older people's sexuality is not only detrimental to their ongoing health and their ability to remain productive into very old age, but it is also an affront to their dignity and a denial of their rights to be sexually active at any age. Structural ageing, changing social mores and increased acceptance of life-long sexuality thus provide the catalyst for the development of sexual health policy addressing the needs of older people (Kirkman, Fox & Dickson-Swift 2016).

References

ABS 2003, *2935.0–Census Paper 03/03–Computer and internet use, 2001*, Population Census Evaluation. Commonwealth of Australia, viewed www.abs.gov.au/AUSSTATS/abs@nsf/DetailsPage/2935.02001?OpenDocument

ABS (Australian Bureau of Statistics) 2011, *8146.0–Household use of information technology, Australia, 2010–11*. Commonwealth of Australia, viewed www.acma.gov.au/~/media/Research%20and%20Analysis/Research/pdf/Australians%20digital%20livesFinal%20pdf.pdf

ACMA (Australian Communications & Media Authority) 2015, *Communications report 2013–14 series Report 1–Australians' digital lives*, March 2015. Commonwealth of Australia, Available at: http://www.acma.gov.au/theACMA/Library/Corporate-library/Corporate-publications/communications-report

Adams, MS, Oye, J, & Parker, TS 2003, 'Sexuality of older adults and the Internet: From sex education to cybersex', *Sexual and Relationship Therapy*, vol. 18, pp. 405–15.

Amin, I 2016, 'Social capital and sexual risk-taking behaviors among older adults in the United States', *Journal of Applied Gerontology*, vol. 35, pp. 982–999.

Anderson, RM 2013, 'Positive sexuality and its impact on overall well-being', *Bundesgesundheitsbl*, vol. 56, pp. 208–14, DOI: 10.1007/s00103-012-1607-z

Association of Progressive Communications 2015, Annual Report. ISBN: 978-92-95102-40-8. Available at: https://www.apc.org/sites/default/files/APC_AnnualReport_2014-web_1.pdf

Averett, P, Yoon, I, & Jenkins, CJ 2012, 'Older lesbian sexuality: Identity, sexual behavior, and the impact of aging', *Journal of Sex Research*, vol. 49, pp. 495–507.

Bach, LE, Mortimer, JA, VandeWeerd, C, & Corvin, J 2014, 'The association of physical and mental health with sexual activity in older adults in a retirement community', *Journal of Sexual Medicine*, vol. 10, no. 11, pp. 2671–8. DOI: 10.1111/jsm.1230

Bateson, DJ, Weisberg, E, McCaffery, KJ, & Luscombe, GM 2012, 'When online becomes offline: Attitudes to safer sex practices in older and younger women using an Australian internet dating service', *Sexual Health*, vol. 9, pp. 152–9.

Beckman, N, Waern, M, Gustafson, D, & Skoog, I 2008, 'Secular trends in self reported sexual activity and satisfaction in Swedish 70 year olds: cross sectional survey of four populations, 1971-2001', British Medical Journal, vol. 337, pp. a279.

Berdychevsky, L, & Nimrod, G 2015, '"Let's talk about sex": Discussions in seniors' online communities', *Journal of Leisure Research*, vol. 47, no. 4, pp. 467–84.

Bisceglio, P 2015, 'Is there love after 30?', *Pacific Standard*, 24 March, viewed 28 December 2015, www.psmag.com/nature-and-technology/tinder-and-the-truth-about-dating-after-30

Brown, SL, & Shinohara, SK 2013, 'Dating relationships in older adulthood: A national portrait', *Journal of Marriage and Family*, vol. 75, pp. 1194–202.

Buchanan, T, & Whitty, MT 2014, 'The online dating romance scam: Causes and consequences of victimhood', *Psychology, Crime & Law*, vol. 20, pp. 261–83.

Burgess, EO 2004, 'Sexuality in midlife and later life couples', in JH Harvey, A Wenzel, & S Sprecher (eds.), *The handbook of sexuality in close relationships*, Lawrence Erlbaum Associates, Mahwah, NJ.

Cali, BE, Coleman, JM, Campbell, C 2013, 'Stranger danger? Women's self-protection intent and the continuing stigma of online dating', *Cyberpsychology, behavior, and social networking*, vol. 16, pp. 853–857.

Carpenter, LM, Nathanson, CA, & Kim, YJ 2006, 'Sex after 40?: Gender, ageism, and sexual partnering in midlife', *Journal of Aging Studies*, vol. 20, pp. 93–106.

Caspi, A, & Gorsky, P 2006, 'Online deception: Prevalence, motivation, and emotion', *Cyber-Psychology & Behavior*, vol. 9, pp. 54–9.

Centers for Disease Control and Prevention 2011, A public health approach for advancing sexual health in the United States: Rationale and options for implementation. Available at: https://www.cdc.gov/sexualhealth/docs/sexualhealthreport-2011-508.pdf

CNN Wire Staff 2011, 'Match.com to begin checking for sex offenders in wake of lawsuit', *CNN*, 18 April, viewed 4 February 2016, www.cnn.com/2011/TECH/web/04/18/match.rape.lawsuit/

Couch, D & Liamputtong, P 2008, 'Online dating and mating: The use of the internet to meet sexual partners', *Qualitative Health Research*, vol. 18, pp. 268–279.

Couch, D, Liamputtong, P, & Pitts, M 2012, 'What are the real and perceived risks and dangers of online dating? Perspectives from online daters', *Health, Risk, & Society*, vol. 14, pp. 697–714.

Cross, C, Smith, RG, & Richards K 2014, 'Challenges of responding to online fraud victimization in Australia', *Trends & Issues in Crime and Criminal Justice*, no. 474, viewed http://eprints.qut.edu.au/72186/1/tandi474.pdf

Daneback, K, Månsson, S-A, Ross, MW, & Markham, CM 2012, 'The internet as a source of information about sexuality', *Sex Education*, vol. 12, pp. 583-98.

Davis, EM, & Fingerman, KL 2016, 'Digital dating: Online profile content of older and younger adults', *Journal of Gerontology: Psychological Sciences*, vol. 71, no. 6, pp. 959–67.

DeFalco, B 2008, 'eHarmony agrees to provide same-sex matches', *The Associated Press*, 20 November, viewed www.nbcnews.com/id/27821393/print/1/displaymode/1098/

DeLamater, J 2012, 'Sexual expression in later life: A review and synthesis', *Journal of Sex Research*, vol. 49, pp. 125–41.

Döring, NM 2009, 'The Internet's impact on sexuality: A critical review of 15 years of research', *Computers in Human Behavior*, vol. 25, pp. 1089–101.

eHarmony 2009, 'Compatible partners website available for gay and lesbian singles seeking long-term relationships', 31 March, viewed 4 February 2016, www.eharmony.com/press-release/19/

eHarmony 2010, 'eHarmony, Inc. settles class action lawsuit over same-sex matching', 26 January, viewed 4 February 2016, www.eharmony.com/press-release/25/

eHarmony 2016, 'Safety tips', viewed 22 July 2016, www.eharmony.com/safe-online-dating/

Experian Hitwise 2012, *Experian marketing services*, viewed www.experian.com.au/blogs/marketing-forward/2012/02/14/data-dating-valentines-day-2012/

Fairfax Digital 2010, RSVP Where more Australians meet. Statistics supplied by RSVP.com Marketing Department July Fairfax Digital, NSW.

Fairfax Media 2010, *RSVP is Australia's number one online dating site*, viewed http://fairfaxmedia.com.au/our-assets/online.dot

Fairfax Digital 2012, *RSVP Date of the Nation Report 2012*. May RSVP.com, Fairfax Digital, NSW.

Fileborn, B, Thorpe, R, Hawkes, G, Minichiello, V, Pitts, M, & Dune, T 2015, 'Sex and the (older) single girl: Experiences of sex and dating in later life', *Journal of Aging Studies*, vol. 33, pp. 67–75.

Finkel, EJ, Eastwick, PW, Karney, BJ, Reis, HT, & Sprecher, S 2012, 'Online dating: A critical analysis from the perspective of psychological science', *Psychological Science in the Public Interest*, vol. 13, pp. 3-66.

Ganong, K, & Larson, E 2011, 'Intimacy and belonging: The association between sexual activity and depression among older adults', *Society & Mental Health*, vol. 1, pp. 153-72.

Global Information Society Watch (GISWatch) 2015, Sexual rights and the Internet. Association for Progressive Communications (APC) and Humanist Institute for Cooperation with Developing Countries (HIVOS). ISBN 978-92-95102-41-5. Available at: https://www.apc.org/sites/default/files/gw2015-full-report_0.pdf

Gott, M 2005, *Sexuality, Sexual Health and Ageing*. Open University Press, Berkshire, UK.

Grimes, GA, Hough MG, Mazur, E, & Signorella, ML 2010, 'Older adults' knowledge of internet hazards', *Educational Gerontology*, vol. 36, pp. 173–92.

Hall, JA, Park, N, Song, H, & Cody, MJ 2010, 'Strategic misrepresentation in online dating: The effects of gender, self-monitoring, and personality traits', *Journal of Social and Personal Relationships*, vol. 27, pp. 117–35.

Hillman, JL 2000, *Clinical perspectives on elderly sexuality*, Kluwer Academic/Plenum Publishers, New York, NY.

Hinchliff, S 2015, 'When it comes to older people and sex, doctors put their heads in the sand', *The Conversation*, June 19, viewed http://theconversation.com/when-it-comes-to-older-people-and-sex-doctors-put-their-heads-in-the-sand-43556

Hinchliff, S, & Gott, M 2004, 'Intimacy, commitment, and adaptation: Sexual relationships within long-term marriages', *Journal of Social and Personal Relationships*, vol. 21, pp. 595–609.

Hogan, B, Li, N, & Dutton, WH 2011, *Me, My Spouse and the Internet*. A global shift in the social relationships of networked individuals: Meeting and dating online comes of age. Oxford Internet Institute (OII), University of Oxford, viewed http://blogs.oii.ox.ac.uk/couples/

Horcher, M 2012, 'World wide web of love, lies, and legislation: Why online dating websites should screen members', *Journal of Computer & Information Law*, vol. 29, pp. 251–78.

Hurd Clarke, L 2006, 'Older women and sexuality: Experiences in marital relationships across the life course', *Canadian Journal on Aging*, vol. 25, pp. 129-40.

Illouz, E 2007, *Cold Intimacies: The Making of Emotional Capitalism*, Polity Press, Cambridge, UK.

Jagger, E 2005, 'Is thirty the new sixty? Dating, age, and gender in a postmodern, consumer society', *Sociology*, vol. 39, pp. 89–106.

Jayson, S 2014, 'Online and mobile dating face privacy, safety concerns', *USA Today*, 27 March, viewed 14 February 2016, www.usatoday.com/story/news/nation/2014/03/27/online-dating-privacy/6957331/

Johnson, AM, Mercer, CH, Erens, B, Copas, A J, McManus, S, Wellings, K, Fenton, KA, Korovessis, C, MacDowall, W, Nanchahal, K, Purdon, S, & Field, J 2001, 'Sexual behavior in Britain: Partnerships, practices, and HIV risk behaviors', *The Lancet*, vol. 358, pp. 1835–1842.

Jönson, H, & Siverskog, A 2012, 'Turning vinegar into wine: Humorous self-presentations among older GLBTQ online daters', *Journal of Aging Studies*, vol. 26, pp. 55–64.

Jorna, P 2016, 'The relationship between age and consumer fraud victimisation', *Trends and Issues in Crime and Criminal Justice*, no. 519, pp. 1–16.

Kirkman, L, Fox, C, & Dickson-Swift, V 2016, 'A case for sexual health policy that includes midlife and older adult sexuality and sexual health', *The International Journal of Aging and Society*, vol. 6, no. 2, 17–27.

Kirkman, L, Kenny, A, & Fox, C 2013, Evidence of absence: Midlife and older adult sexual health policy in Australia, *Sexuality Research and Social Policy*, vol. 10, pp. 135-48.

Kontual, O, & Haavio-Mannila, E 2009, 'The impact of aging on human sexual activity and sexual desire', *Journal of Sex Research*, vol. 46, pp. 46–56.

Laumann, EO, Paik, A, & Rosen, RC 1999, 'Sexual dysfunction in the United States: Prevalence and predictors', *JAMA*, vol. 281, pp. 537–544.

Laumann, EO, Paik, A, Glasser, DB, Kang, J-H, Wang, T, Levinson, B, Moreira, ED, Nicolosi, A, & Gingell, C 2006, 'A cross-national study of subjective well-being among older women and men: Findings from the global study of sexual attitudes and behaviors', *Archives of Sexual Behavior*, vol. 35, pp. 145–61.

Lindau, ST, Schumm, LP, Laumann, EO, Levinson, W, O'Muircheartaigh, CA, & Waite, LJ 2007, 'A study of sexuality and health among older adults in the United States', *The New England Journal of Medicine*, vol. 357, pp. 762–74.

Lyons, A, Pitts, M, Grierson, J, Thorpe, R, & Power, J 2010, 'Ageing with HIV: health and psychosocial well-being of older gay men', *AIDS Care*, vol. 22, pp. 1236-44.

Malta, S 2007, 'Love actually! Older adults and their romantic Internet relationships', *Australian Journal of Emerging Technologies & Society*, vol. 5, pp. 84–102.

Malta, S 2013, *Love, sex and intimacy in new late-life romantic relationships*. Doctoral thesis, August 2013. Swinburne University, Hawthorn, VIC. Download via Research Bank, viewed http://researchbank.swinburne.edu.au/vital/access/manager/Repository/swin:3 5671?queryType=vitalDismax&query=Love%2C+sex+and+intimacy+in+new+late-life +romantic+relationships&y=0&x=0

Malta, S, & Farquharson, K 2014, 'The initiation and progression of late-life romantic relationships', *Journal of Sociology*, vol. 50, pp. 237–51.

Match.com 2016, *Good advice–safety tips to follow*, viewed 21 July 2016, www.match.com/help/safetytips.aspx

McFarlane, L, & Bocij, P 2003, 'An exploration of predatory behavior in cyberspace: Towards a typology of cyberstalkers', *First Monday*, vol. 8, no. 9, np. viewed http://journals.uic.edu/ojs/index.php/fm/article/view/1076/996

McFarlane, M, Kachur, R, Bull, S, & Rietmeijer, C 2004, 'Women, the internet, and sexually transmitted infections', *Journal of Women's Health*, vol. 13, pp. 689–94.

McIntosh, WD, Locker, L, Jr, Briley, K, Ryan, R, & Scott, AJ 2011, 'What do older adults seek in their potential romantic partners? Evidence from online personal ads', *International Journal of Aging and Human Development*, vol. 72, pp. 67–82.

McWilliams, S, & Barrett, AE 2014, 'Online dating in middle and later life: Gendered expectations and experiences', *Journal of Family Issues*, vol. 35, pp. 411–36.

Minichiello, V, Hawkes, G, & Pitts, M 2011, 'HIV, sexually transmitted infections, and sexuality in later life', *Current Infectious Diseases Report*, vol. 13, pp. 182–7.

Minichiello, V, Plummer, D, & Macklin, M 2003, 'Sex in Australia: Older Australians do it too!', *Australian and New Zealand Journal of Public Health*, vol. 27, no. 4, pp. 466–7.

Nash, P, Willis, P, Tales, A, & Cryer, T 2015, 'Sexual health and sexual activity in later life', *Reviews in Clinical Gerontology*, vol. 25, pp. 22–30.

Nicolosi, A, Laumann, EO, Glasser, DB, Moreira, ED, Paik, A, & Gingell, C 2004, 'Sexual behavior and sexual dysfunctions after age 40: The global study of sexual attitudes and behaviors', *Adult Urology*, vol. 64, pp. 991–7.

Novak, M 2016, *Issues in Aging*. 3rd Edition, Routledge, New York, NY.

Orel, NA, Spence, M, & Steele, J 2005, 'Getting the message out to older adults: Effective HIV health education risk reduction publications', *The Journal of Applied Gerontology*, vol. 24, pp. 490–508.

Orel, NA, Wright, JM, & Wagner, J 2004, 'Scarcity of HIV/AIDS risk-reduction materials targeting the needs of older adults among state departments of public health', *The Gerontologist*, vol. 44, pp. 693–6.

Perrin, A, & Duggan, M 2015, *Americans' internet access 2000–2015*, Pew Research Center, Washington, DC, 26 June, viewed 2 February 2016 www.pewinternet.org/files/2015/06/2015–06–26_internet-usage-across-demographics-discover_FINAL.pdf

Pittaro, ML 2007, 'Cyber stalking: An analysis of online harassment and intimidation', *International Journal of Cyber Criminology*, vol. 1, pp. 180–97.

Potârcă, G, Mills, M, & Neberich, W 2015, 'Relationship preferences among gay and lesbian online daters: Individual and contextual influences', *Journal of Marriage and Family*, vol. 77, pp. 523–41.

PR Newswire 2016, *Match Releases New Study on LGBTQ Single Population*. May 24, viewed www.prnewswire.com/news/match

Rege, A 2009, 'What's love got to do with it? Exploring online dating scams and identity fraud', *International Journal of Cyber Crime*, vol. 3, pp. 494–512.

Richters J & Rissel C 2005, *Doing it Down Under: The Sexual Lives of Australians*. Allen & Unwin, Sydney, NSW.

Rosen, RC, & Bachmann, GA 2008, 'Sexual well-being, happiness, and satisfaction, in women: The case for a new conceptual paradigm', *Journal of Sex and Marital Therapy*, vol. 34, pp. 291–297.

Rosenbloom, S 2010, 'New online-date detectives can unmask Mr. or Ms. wrong', *The New York Times*, 18 December, viewed 4 February 2016 www.nytimes.com/2010/12/19/us/19date.html?_r=0

Rosenfeld, MJ, & Thomas, RJ 2012, 'Searching for a mate: The rise of the internet as a social intermediary', *American Sociological Review*, vol. 77, pp. 523–47.

Rowntree, MR 2014, '"Comfortable in my own skin": A new form of sexual expression for ageing baby boomers', *Journal of Aging Studies*, vol. 31, pp. 150–8.

Sanders, S 2015, 'Tinder's premium dating app will cost you more if you're older', *NPR All Tech Considered*, 2 March, viewed 28 December www.npr.org/sections/alltechconsidered/2015/03/02/390236051/tinders-premium-dating-app-will-cost-you-more-if-youre-older

Scaunich, S, 2014, *The sexual health of women aged 50 and over: A literature review*. Women's Health in the South-East (WHISE), Bishop H, & Bugden M (eds.). Available at: http://www.whise.org.au/assets/docs/whise_info/The%20sexual%20health%20of%20women%20aged%2050%20and%20over.%20A%20Literature%20Review.pdf

Schick, V, Herbenick, D, Reece, M, Sanders, SA, Dodge, B, Middlestadt, SE, & Fortenberry, DJ 2010, 'Sexual behaviors, condom use, and sexual health of Americans over 50: Implications for sexual health promotion for older adults', *Journal of Sexual Medicine*, vol. 7, pp. 315–29.

Sherrard, J, & Wainwright, E 2013, 'Sexually transmitted infections in older men', *Maturitas*, vol. 74, pp. 203–5.

Sontag, S 1972, 'The double standard of aging', *Saturday Review of the Society*, September 23, pp. 29–38.

Stephure, RJ, Boon, SD, MacKinnon, SL, & Deveau, VL 2009, 'Internet initiated relationships: Associations between age and involvement in online dating', *Journal of Computer-Mediated Communication*, vol. 14, pp. 658–81.

Stone, A 2011, 'Match.com to begin checking users against sex offender database', *ABC News*, 18 April, viewed 3 February 2016, http://abcnews.go.com/US/match-begin-checking-users-sex-offender-database/story?id=13396930

Toma, CL, Hancock, JT, & Ellison, NB 2008, 'Separating fact from fiction: An examination of deceptive self-presentation in online dating profiles', *Personality and Social Psychology Bulletin*, vol. 34, pp. 1023–36.

Wada, M, Clarke LH, & Rozanova, J 2015, 'Constructions of sexuality in later life: Analyses of Canadian magazine and newspaper portrayals of online dating', *Journal of Aging Studies*, vol. 32, pp. 40–9.

Watson, WK, & Stelle, C 2011, 'Dating for older women: Experiences and meanings of dating in later life', *Journal of Women & Aging*, vol. 23, pp. 263–75.

Whitty, MT, & Buchanan, T 2012, 'The online romance scam: A serious cybercrime', *Cyberpsychology, Behavior, and Social Networking*, vol. 15, pp. 181–4.

Whitty, MT, & Carr, A 2006, *Cyberspace romance: The psychology of online relationships*, Palgrave Macmillan, Hampshire, UK.

Woloski-Wruble, AC, Oliel, Y, LeefsMa, M, & Hochner-Celnikier, D 2010, 'Sexual activities, sexual and life satisfaction, and successful aging in women', *Journal of Sexual Medicine*, vol. 7, pp. 2401–10.

World Health Organisation (WHO) 2015, *Sexual health, human rights and the law*, WHO Document Production Services, Geneva, Switzerland.

Zeiss, AM, & Kasl-Godley, J 2001, 'Sexuality in older adults' relationships', *Generations*, vol. 25, pp. 18–25.

12

CONCLUSION

Moving forward, implementing change

Sharron Hinchliff and Catherine Barrett

Introduction

In this final chapter we draw together the conclusions and recommendations made in the preceding chapters to address the challenges that come from asserting and implementing the sexual rights of older people. Edited collections of this type often do not have concluding chapters. However, given the significant lack of recognition of the sexual rights of older people and the need to change this situation, we believe it is important to have such a chapter to build on what we already know and to suggest ways forward.

The authors of each chapter have demonstrated why a sexual rights framework for older people is needed now. In many countries, older people are marginalised and subjected to damaging prejudice and discrimination based on their age. And when being 'old' intersects with other social categories that are in the minority, such as sexual orientation, gender identity, and race, older people can be further marginalised. Calasanti and Slevin (2006) point out that marginalisation has serious consequences for people's chances in later life: when individuals are 'perceived to be old' they lose power, which opens them up to exploitation, abuse, and the many inequalities deemed 'natural, and thus beyond dispute' (Calasanti & Slevin 2006, p. 6). There is no doubt that ageism is pervasive and taken for granted so much so that it tends to go unnoticed. Indeed, it has been argued that negative ageism is 'socially-condoned' (e.g. North & Fiske 2012), in that it is more prevalent, and less challenged, than racism and sexism. According to *Age International*, there is firm evidence that while instances of racism and sexism are declining, cases of ageism are increasing (Age International 2017).

A sexual rights framework for older people aims to ensure that all older people are treated with dignity and respect and are able to influence the direction of their lives through the choices they make. A sexual rights framework should protect, yet guarantee access to, these choices. A sexual rights framework for older people should also acknowledge that sexuality is influenced by life experiences. As Heidari (2016, p. 3) has argued, a culmination of many factors, including 'poverty, marginalisation, violence, harmful practices such as female genital mutilation and child marriage, or poor reproductive health', require examination if we are to expand our awareness of healthy sexual ageing.

The chapters presented in this collection are some examples of the application of a sexual rights framework for older people. Each has been built around the ethos of sexual rights and has directly addressed at least one of the sexual rights presented in Chapter 2. Indeed, all the chapters covered Right 1: the right to equality and non-discrimination, as the right to being treated without prejudice and discrimination underpins the whole premise of this book. Many chapters covered the right to life, liberty, and security (Right 2) by, for example, drawing attention to the ways that people who engage in non-conforming sexual behaviours, or have diverse sexual orientations or gender identities, can face threats to life, freedom, and personal safety. The right to autonomy and bodily integrity (Right 3) was covered by authors who explored issues ranging from the societal messages about the sexuality of older people to the body-changing procedures of gender transition. Indeed, because sexuality is closely linked with power and politics, the basic right to make choices about our own bodies is required in order for most other human rights to be attainable (Runeborg & Anderson 2010).

Our relationships with other people, from interpersonal (intimate, familial) to social (friendships, social networks, communities), have been central to this book, and some authors discussed the degrading treatment that older people can experience in connection with their age and/or sexuality (Right 4: the right to be free from torture and cruel, inhumane or degrading treatment or punishment). This included the ways that older people are approached and responded to by health and social professionals who lack awareness, understanding, and/or the skills to support the diverse sexualities of older people. Indeed, not all health professionals and service providers are aware that sexual rights can and should be applied to older people, thus unintentional violations occur.

When discussing gender-based violence and older women, Cooper and Crocket (2015, p. 59) indicate that 'it is not uncommon for health professionals working with older adults to accept alternative explanations for injuries that would be clearly attributed to sexual trauma among younger patients'. Indeed, Chapter 8, dealt with the sexual assault of older women, and most directly addressed sexual Right 5, the right to be free from all forms of violence and coercion as related to sex, sexual orientation, and gender identity, even though it was noted in many other chapters. The right to privacy (Right 6) was implicit throughout all the chapters but, as pointed out in Chapter 2, there is a line that may be crossed by well-meaning service providers who move towards LGBTI inclusive care and practice: privacy may be unintentionally breached through the storage and sharing of personal data. Indeed, services should help older people to reach the highest attainable level of sexual health and well-being (Right 7), and in order to do this, protection from prejudice and discrimination is paramount.

The right to sexual pleasure runs throughout this book and fits with the WAS Declaration of Sexual Rights, described in Chapter 2, which is underpinned by a principle of pleasure. However, we should recognise the diverse ways that older people obtain sexual pleasure and, as noted in Chapter 1, that not all older people have a desire to be sexually active. Scientific progress and its application (Right 8) moves beyond pharmaceutical treatments for age-related sexual 'dysfunctions', which formed the core of Chapter 10, to the development of medicines to improve health and well-being and control disease. Such developments can, in turn, have a beneficial impact on interpersonal relationships and older people's sexuality. This links closely with the right to information that is scientifically accurate and applicable to diverse groups (Right 9). Scientifically accurate information is missing for many older people, for example, a lack of information on the risks associated with unprotected sex – as pointed out in Chapter 9 – which can play a part in the spread of sexually transmitted infections (STIs). Scientific information may be misconstrued by the popular media. For example, the stories we read in newspapers and magazines tend to present the message that Viagra and other sexuopharmaceuticals can 'save' the sex lives of older men by maintaining their erections, as though it is a magic pill, while failing to mention that it does not work for all men, and for many causes a long-lasting, painful headache that prevents them from using the drug again. Again, the right to comprehensive sexuality education (Right 10) is a feature of the book overall, with many authors making the point that sex education is lacking for older people and the staff and service providers who are part of aged care. Comprehensive sexual education can serve to inform older people, family members, and those whose work brings them into contact with older people, about the existence of sexual rights, what the sexual rights are, and how they can be upheld.

Taking steps to improve the sexual rights of older people can help improve their living conditions by promoting healthy relationships and empowering people to take action. Relationships, as above, have formed a thread throughout the chapters in this collection, and the right to enter and leave interpersonal relationships (Right 11) may not be a clear or easy option for some people. For example, those in abusive relationships may have restricted movement due to the level of control and coercion in the relationship. Those in aged care facilities may lose the right to form new intimate relationships, as their own family or care staff may disapprove. Furthermore, the idea about what is an 'acceptable' intimate relationship shifts over time and place, and many Western countries have witnessed a rise in midlife marital divorces and increased opportunities for 'new' types of relationships (e.g. same-sex marriage).

The right to freedom of expression and thought (Right 12) was directly addressed in the chapters that discussed older people as not 'fitting' the norms, ideals, and expectations of old age, gender, and sexuality, so chiefly Chapters 3 and 4, which made reference to older women and older men and the 'sexy oldie'. This right can be even more restricted for people who identify as LGBTI, as Chapters 5, 6, and 7 demonstrated. Similarly, the right to freedom of association and peaceful assembly (Right 13) is perhaps most evident in the chapters discussing sexual practices or characteristics that have been (and still are in some contexts) deemed socially unacceptable. The right to participation in public and political life (Right 14) is advocated by all chapter authors and forms a central premise of this book. As we discuss later in this chapter, the perspectives of older people should be utilised to inform and develop policy that is aimed at improving the lives and care of older people. And similarly, Right 15, the right to access justice, remedies, and redress, cuts through the whole of the book.

In the remaining sections of this chapter, we outline our key messages before moving on to the recommendations for practice, policy-making, research, and activism. We describe strategies for raising awareness of the sexual rights of older people by including critical sexuality studies and participatory action research to build evidence around rights violations and to engage communities in debating and constructing strategies for reform. And we end with a 'call to action': none of the suggested changes will come into place without the sustained efforts of people who have a passion for addressing the inequalities experienced by older people.

Key messages

The key messages we turn to now are not presented hierarchically; we believe that each is important in its own right. And while they interlink, some may need to be in place before others can be implemented. We recognise that there will be different starting points for individuals and organisations who are taking steps to change the sexual rights landscape, and that this will be influenced by time and place. The values of a society are always influential, and socially accepted norms will play a role in what part(s) of this sexual rights framework is adopted and when. Throughout this book, sexualities have been understood as the 'result of diverse social practices that give meaning to human activities, of social definitions and self-definitions, of struggles between those who have power to define and regulate, and those who resist' (Weeks 2011, pp. 204–5). And thus, following Foucault (1978), we acknowledge the influence of governing bodies and disciplinary institutions in the surveillance of sexuality. We simply cannot escape the politics of where we are located.

Key message 1: acknowledge the sexual agency and identity of older people

Over the past two decades, sexual rights have begun to be applied broadly, moving away from a sole focus upon young heterosexuals and the reproductive context. Lesbian and gay activism has helped shift the focus to the sexual rights of LGBTI communities, and feminism played an influential role in driving attention towards women and other marginalised groups, including those categorised as having low socio-economic status. Unfortunately, the view that sexual rights should apply to all does not exist in all countries today, a position that many – including the authors of this book – are working hard to change. Acknowledging the sexual agency of older people is the first step we can take towards promoting social change and consequently improving the support and resources available so that older people's sexual rights can be achieved. Acknowledging sexual agency requires us to challenge the stereotypes about sex and (older) age, which place older people as exempt from, or disinterested in, sexuality. Recognising and raising awareness of the sexual rights of older people will also require that we view older people as full citizens. Older people who assert their sexual rights are asserting their right to exist.

Key message 2: move beyond the biomedical assumptions

We need to move beyond the narrow biomedical assumptions about older people and sexuality. It seems that assumptions made about young people's experiences and needs are often applied to older people without any consideration of what older people themselves think or what they deem as important. We know, for example, that sexual activity tends to be broadly defined by older people, and as it can be important to quality of life, sexual pleasure may be gained from intimacy more than actual physical activity (Bouman 2013; Waite et al. 2009; Wentzell 2013). We need to be wary of frameworks that, for example, equate sexual desirability with young (particularly female) bodies, or associate sexual pleasure with an erect penis, as the authors in this book have argued. Presenting (a narrow version of) sexual desirability as something that can be attained through the consumption of products and consistent engagement in beauty practices neglects the influence of health status, income, and cultural context. And presenting an erect penis as the pinnacle of sexual pleasure negates the experiences of those who derive pleasure and satisfaction from a broad range of sexual activities. In moving forward, we also must be mindful that we do not create more stereotypes along the way. For example, that older people can be considered 'sexy' *only* if they dress a certain way and have particular physical characteristics, such as a slim physique, a wrinkle-free face, and an able body (Hinchliff & Gott 2016; Hurd Clarke 2010). And, thus, where sexiness, as defined with reference to young people, is applied to those who are much older. Additional potential stereotypes that we ought to be aware of, and avoid generating, is that all older people *want* to be sexually active, would like the option to use sexual technologies (e.g. Viagra), or that they must be sexually active if they are to 'age well'.

This is why it is important to hear and respond to what older people have to say about their experiences. Biomedical frameworks can be significantly progressed by social science research in order to influence the development of health care and health policy in ways that reflect the realities of older people's lives. Such progression is a key message of this book.

Key message 3: recognise diversity

Achieving the sexual rights of older people requires recognition that older people are not a homogenous group. Older people are diverse in terms of the values and beliefs they hold, and other factors such as their own life experiences, sexual orientation, gender identity, ethnicity, and socioeconomic status. The application of a sexual rights framework cannot be done in a way that is prescriptive: it requires a flexible vision, with recognition that there is no 'one size fits all' approach. To be mindful of the varied ways that sexuality is understood and experienced, both across and within cultures, cannot be underestimated. Assumptions of heterosexuality continue to be made by health and social professionals, despite the wider recognition of diverse sexual identities (Cronin & King 2010). The concept of human rights is not detached from the politics within the culture it sits, and we need to carefully consider whose interests a particular rights-based approach serves (e.g. when a governing body fails to recognise and support any sexual orientation that is not heterosexual). This takes us to our next key message: that we must be aware of, make reference to, and act upon power and privilege.

Key message 4: be alert to power and privilege

Indeed, the language that we use to describe people, their actions, and the social categories they belong to can be powerful in shaping our views or persuading us to accept a specific outlook. Language gains prominence when it is accompanied (spoken or written) by individuals or institutions that are deemed to have authority, as the status of 'expert' legitimates their words. Experts come in many forms, and we should be sensitive to experts who are community leaders and those who uphold cultural 'laws'. Scientists and clinicians in Western cultures are in a position where their opinions are viewed as credible and rarely challenged, and this is particularly apparent in the area of sexuality. Influenced by the work of Foucault, Ussher and Baker (1993, p. 1) assert that sexuality has 'always been conceptualised as a potential problem', one that is regulated by the distinction between 'normal' (healthy) and 'abnormal' (unhealthy) sexuality. This distinction has applied both to the sexual behaviours we engage in and the sexual partners we choose.

An issue to consider here is the extent to which expert, scientific, and medical regimes of knowledge penetrate an individual's self-perceptions and influence their behaviour. As Nicolson (1993, p. 57) has argued, 'knowledge derives from power and that knowledge reproduces itself through the social mechanisms of norm-setting which in turn have a psychological dimension; that is, they penetrate self-cognitions'. When medical or religious discourses pathologise or imply abnormality in some other way, it is no surprise that the people they purport to describe can experience distress. Pathologising language not only serves to blame individuals for their behaviours, but it also licenses experts to talk about the matter. As McLaren (2005, p. 4) has argued, we must 'keep in mind that by privileging the official discourse there is the danger of ignoring those that could not be so freely expressed'.

Examples have been provided throughout this book of the ways that older people are talked about which associates them with powerlessness, weakness, and dependency. Ageist discourses can intersect with other damaging discourses, influencing the ways that older people are viewed and treated within societies. Again, we must ask in whose interests this form of ageism serves – it privileges the young and disempowers the old. Alternatively, discourses that accompany the concept of 'successful ageing' at first glance appear to be positive; they celebrate being old and what older people can achieve. However, within a neoliberal framework where the expectation is to age healthily and independently and thus *be* the 'virtuous citizen', it is limited to older people who have physical ability, and the required social and material resources of support. Older people in poor health may find it difficult, if indeed possible, to exercise regularly, to maintain social relationships, and so on, yet the responsibility for good health sits firmly on their shoulders. The concepts of 'active ageing', 'successful ageing', and 'positive ageing' can be problematic for the expectations they create and the people they exclude.

Recommendations

We believe that the above interlinking messages will help individuals and organisations to address the key themes of invisibility, silencing, prejudice, discrimination, and lack of understanding that have emerged from the chapters as a whole. We now offer suggestions about some of the ways that this sexual rights framework for older people can be utilised. Relevant to all the messages above is that older people should be central to discussions about, and decisions made, regarding their sexual rights. Involving older people in this way will allow user-focused agendas to be established, the most appropriate needs to be met, and be effective in challenging prejudice and instigating change. Furthermore, it will help older people to update or develop their sexual literacy, if required. Although the book has focused predominantly on people aged 65 and older, we recognise that there may be differences between those who are young-old (aged 65–79 years) and those who are old-old (aged 80+).[1]

Awareness-raising

Raising public awareness about an issue requires a campaign that contains a specific message or set of messages. Its aim should be to help people, policy-makers, service providers, and relevant communities to understand the topic at hand. Such campaigns are most effective if they are perceived by the public to have relevance to their lives. They must also be culturally sensitive. Awareness-raising campaigns for the sexual rights of older people could utilise older people's narratives to help with recognition of the campaigns. They could anchor themselves on relationships (intimate, interpersonal, social, familial), which are a central feature of all of our lives. The campaigns could employ various means of communication, including articles in newspapers, features in magazines, programmes on television, posters in appropriate public areas such as clinic waiting rooms, and interviews on the radio. Technology has changed the sexualities and sexual health arena, and social media is useful to spread messages to a global audience. A pre-planned coordinated strategy that is large scale, has a long life, and is culturally sensitive would be most effective.

Developing knowledge and skills

Combining activism with education can raise public awareness in a powerful way. Education, whether formal or informal, can help older people to acquire knowledge and develop skills to communicate effectively about their sexual rights. Indeed, access to education and information can support people to make informed decisions about their sexuality and to protect their health and well-being, and is therefore associated with positive health outcomes (WHO 2015a p. 2). As outlined in Chapter 2, older people have the right to access comprehensive information regarding their sexuality, and the development of knowledge and skills should focus on older people as a priority. As indicated previously, this information needs to be scientifically accurate. The World Health Organization points out that it should not be censored, withheld, or intentionally misrepresented by the governing state (WHO 2015b).

Health inequalities can build up across the life-course, providing a cumulative disadvantage for older people (WHO 2015a), which must be borne in mind. For example, today's generation of older LGBTI people may fear reproach from health and social care professionals due to their historical experiences of homophobic or transphobic abuse. For professionals, having an understanding of gender socialisation and the ways that it can influence their thinking will be of benefit. This could include learning about implicit bias, where we discriminate against people based on social categories such as race or gender even though we do not believe ourselves to be prejudiced, and how that can come into play in our interactions with others. While interventions aimed at individuals and groups have been shown to be effective in tackling implicit bias (see, for example, Devine et al. 2012), a broader approach is still required where a social responsibility to tackle such prejudice is in place.

Education and training should provide a safe space for health and social professionals to explore their own values and what this may mean for their own professional practice. This can include enhanced communication skills training to tackle the sensitive and unknown, and to help reduce any discomfort they feel around sexuality, particularly around older people's sexuality. Research has shown that students with more knowledge of older people's sexuality were more tolerant towards it (Adana et al. 2015) and more willing to assess sexual health (Flaget-Greener, Gonzalez & Sprankle 2015). To help health and social professionals apply what they have learned, and ensure that the knowledge they have gained does not stay in the teaching room, practical resources that enable change and improvement should coexist with the training materials. We now look at what can be done here, in terms of providing relevant, comprehensive, and up-to-date policy in this area.

Informing policy and establishing protocols

It is clear that policies which support the sexual rights of older people need to be in place both locally and nationally. Policies already exist in many countries, such as sexual health frameworks, but they do not always take a life-course approach and include older people. This can easily be remedied. Institutions and organisations would benefit from utilising their own sexual rights policy. Resource kits developed for aged care services that include tools as well as policies have been very well received in Australia, and they can be modified to fit the requirements of individual services.[2]

Older people who are being cared for by family or service providers need to feel safe, and it is imperative that they can trust their carer(s). This is a concern for *all* older people, not only those who may be vulnerable to sexual assault due to cognitive decline, or those who fear the repercussions of openly disclosing their sexual orientation or gender identity. It is crucial that we create cultures and environments that are inclusive and respectful of the diversity of older people. This requires an approach that combats not only ageism but also sexism, homophobia, and transphobia. The World Health Organization (2015) points out that people whose 'consensual sexual behaviour' is considered a criminal offence may hide their behaviours from health and social professionals due to stigmatization, but also from a fear of arrest and prosecution, which can deter them from accessing services in the first place. Such barriers to seeking and receiving care can exacerbate current health issues and result in serious health problems.

Promoting and protecting the sexual rights of older people includes providing avenues for people, including older people themselves, to report rights violations in a way that does not risk their safety. Equality could be added as a fixed item to the agendas of meetings, and be made central to the discussions people have, when relevant, in the workplace. We can help to create appropriate resources and policy by identifying the gaps in existing policy and offering ideas to fill them. This takes us to the next recommendation: addressing the language of inequality.

Addressing the language of inequality

As stated earlier, language is powerful so it is imperative that we pay attention to the ways that older people, and their health and well-being, are talked about and described. Written and verbal language may need to be adjusted so that it does not reinforce negative stereotypes of older people and instead normalises the sexual rights of older people. A simple step, and possibly a starting point, is to check that the language used in key documents (e.g. policy) is non-discriminatory; that is, free from potentially damaging connotations about older people based on their age and other social categories they belong to. Negative stereotypes about older people are implicit in many Western societies, and because of this they often go unnoticed.

Part of addressing the language of inequality, and implementing many of the recommendations outlined above, includes presenting information about the positive aspects of older people's sexuality. Much of the research conducted to date and the available literature focuses on the negative aspects of sex, sexuality, and ageing (e.g., the sexual 'dysfunctions' that can come with age, or the challenges that older people face when they start an intimate relationship while living in long-term care). While it is important to highlight and respond to such issues, as many authors within this book have done, it is also imperative to celebrate ageing. Positive representations (without creating expectations that older people cannot live up to) could help to tackle the stigma and taboo that currently surround the sexual rights of older people.

Conclusion

The foregoing suggestions are not exhaustive. We expect that people will identify further recommendations in relation to their own needs and those of their environment. We encourage all with an interest in the sexual rights of older people to share the recommendations in the spirit of congeniality, as they tackle the inequalities that many older people face. Collective action is key to progress. Thus, we believe it is necessary to take a multi-pronged approach to promoting the sexual rights of older people, and to engage with older people, community groups, voluntary sector organisations, activists, as well as the main providers of health and social care. Engaging with communities of older people can help break down stereotypes. From an intergenerational perspective, when children and young people mix with old people, it to helps provide a sense of shared identity, to increase trust, and to foster a respect for differences (WHO 2015a).

Where individuals are located in the world will influence how they can progress the sexual rights of older people. While states are obliged to ensure their laws and regulations around sexual health align with human rights laws and standards (WHO 2015b), a statement released by the Scientific and Technical Advisory Group and Gender Rights Advisory Panel, which sits within the United Nations, points to a growing resistance to the 'promotion, protection and fulfilment of sexual and reproductive health rights' around the world (2017, p. 1). If sexual rights in general are at risk, it could make it more difficult to implement the sexual rights of older people, as their needs are rarely considered as part of a sexual rights agenda.

But we can all do something. Start small if necessary, give talks, write, develop resources and share them, and make connections with relevant people, communities, and organisations. Grow so that you have local, national, and international spread. The key is to be active, to participate, and to get your message heard. A majority of this work requires changing social attitudes to encourage the recognition of the sexual rights of older groups. We can all be advocates and create change.

Questions will be asked as to whether it is best to approach sexual rights from a life-course perspective, as applied to all regardless of age, or to look at the sexual rights of people per se, separated out from younger age groups. The advantage of taking a life-course approach is that it does not perpetuate and reinforce the traditional view that sexual rights apply chiefly to young people, but such a holistic approach may not suit all attempts at promotion of, and activism around, the sexual rights of older people. Institutions and individuals should choose the approach that best suits their needs and the local and national environments, and thus be culturally sensitive. Indeed, human rights tend to be approached from a life-course perspective, and while they are divisible by age, how this is interpreted by individuals and institutions will, of course, always vary.

The sexual rights framework for older people presented in this book can be adapted to suit disease, disability, and HIV: areas that were not fully covered in this collection. As stated previously, it forms just one version of a sexual rights approach. It is clear that more research needs to be carried out, with regard to topics and in terms of geographical location. Ways forward include researching the sexual rights of older people in middle- and low-income countries, which would not only help build an evidence base, but it would assist communities to learn from each other. We end this chapter with the words of Anna Runeborg and Christina Anderson (2010, p. 4) that 'sexual rights are important for everyone, irrespective of gender, age, ethnicity or sexual identity'. They warn that sexual rights can be perceived as a threat to tradition by religious and political institutions, and they recommend that we 'demystify' what it means to fulfil people's sexual rights. Part of the process of clarifying our understanding about sexual rights is to ensure that leaders are fully informed about which changes are required, why they are required, and the benefits they, and their communities, will see from such changes.

Notes

1 We acknowledge that these categories of old age can be in themselves influenced by subjective age, as well as the physical and mental health indicators of age.
2 Examples of a sexual well-being and safety policy, and a sexual boundaries policy, can be seen from the following link: www.opalinstitute.org/tools.html

References

Adana, F, Arslantaş, H, Abacigil, F, Cabuk, M, Cetinkaya, S & Demir, O 2015, Knowledge and attitudes of a group of university students toward sexuality in aged people, *Studiu Original JMB*, vol. 1, pp. 38–40.

Age International 2017, *What is ageism?* Viewed 4 March 2017, www.ageinternational.org. uk/what-we-do/Policy-where-we-stand-/ageism/

Bouman, WP 2013, 'Sexuality in later life', in T Dening & A Thomas (eds.), *The Oxford textbook of old age psychiatry*, Oxford University Press, Oxford.

Calasanti, TM & Slevin, KF 2006, 'Introduction: Age matters', in TM Calasanti & KF Slevin (eds.), *Age matters: Realigning feminist thinking*, Routledge, New York.

Cooper, B & Crockett, C 2015, Gender-based violence and HIV across the life course: Adopting a sexual rights framework to include older women, *Reproductive Health Matters*, vol. 23, no. 46, pp. 56–61.

Cronin, A & King, A 2010, Power, inequality and identification: Exploring diversity and intersectionality amongst older LGB adults, *Sociology*, vol. 44, no. 5, pp. 876–892.

Devine, PG, Forscher, PS, Austin, AJ & Cox, WT 2012, Long-term reduction in implicit race bias: A prejudice habit-breaking intervention, *Journal of Experimental Social Psychology*, vol. 48, no. 6, pp. 1267–1278.

Flaget-Greener, M, Gonzalez, CA & Sprankle, E 2015, Are sociodemographic characteristics, education and training, and attitudes toward older adults' sexuality predictive of willingness to assess sexual health in a sample of US psychologists? *Sexual & Relationship Therapy*, vol. 30, no. 1, pp. 10–24.

Foucault, M 1978, *The history of sexuality: An introduction*, Pantheon Books, New York.

Heidari, S 2016, Sexuality and older people: A neglected issue, *Reproductive Health Matters*, vol. 24, no. 48, pp. 1–5.

Hinchliff, S & Gott, M 2016, 'Ageing and sexuality in Western societies: Changing perspectives on sexual activity, sexual expression, and the sexy older body', in E Peel & R Harding (eds.), *Ageing and sexualities: Interdisciplinary perspectives*, Ashgate/Routledge, London.

Hurd Clarke, L 2010, *Facing age: Women growing older in anti-aging culture*, Rowman & Littlefield Publishers, Plymouth, UK.

McLaren, A 2005, *Twentieth-century sexuality: A history*, Blackwell, Malden, MA.

Nicolson, P 1993, 'Public values and private beliefs: Why do women refer themselves for sex therapy?', in JM Ussher & CD Baker (eds.), *Psychological perspectives on sexual problems: New directions in theory and practice*, Routledge, London.

North, MS & Fiske, ST 2012, An inconvenienced youth? Ageism and its potential intergenerational roots, *Psychological Bulletin*, vol. 138, no. 5, p. 982.

Programme of Research, Development and Research Training in Human Reproduction, viewed 19 March 2017, www.who.int/reproductivehealth/en/

Runeborg, A & Anderson, C 2010, *Sexual rights for all: Swedish International Development cooperation Agency (SIDA)*, viewed 29 August 2015, www.sida.se/globalassets/global/about-sida/sa-arbetar-vi/sexual-rights-for-all_webb.pdf

Scientific and Technical Advisory Group and Gender Rights Advisory Panel 2017, *Statement on the promotion, protection and fulfilment of sexual and reproductive health rights*. United Nations system, the UNDP/UNFPA/UNICEF/WHO/World Bank Special.

Ussher, JM & Baker, CD 1993, 'Sexuality: Whose problem?', in JM Ussher & CD Baker (eds.), *Psychological perspectives on sexual problems: New directions in theory and practice*, Routledge, London.

Waite, LJ, Laumann, EO, Das, A & Schumm, LP 2009, Sexuality: Measures of partnerships, practices, attitudes, and problems in the national social life, health, and aging study, *The Journals of Gerontology Series B: Psychological Sciences and Social Sciences*, vol. 64, pp. i56–i66.

Weeks, J 2011, *The languages of sexuality*. Routledge, Oxon, UK.

Wentzell, EA 2013, *Maturing masculinities: Aging, chronic illness, and viagra in Mexico*, Duke University Press, Durham, NC.

World Health Organization 2015a, *World report on ageing and health*, viewed 01 March 2017, http://apps.who.int/iris/bitstream/10665/186463/1/9789240694811_eng.pdf?ua=1

World Health Organization 2015b, Sexual health, human rights and the law, World Health Organization, viewed 20 December 2016, http://apps.who.int/iris/handle/10665/175556

INDEX

Note: Page numbers in bold indicate a table on the corresponding page.